Acid Alkaline Companion

An Accompaniment to Herman Aihara's *Acid and Alkaline*

by Carl Ferré

George Ohsawa Macrobiotic Foundation
Chico, California

Other Books by Carl Ferré
Pocket Guide to Macrobiotics
Compiler of *Essential Ohsawa*

Cover design by Carl Campbell
Editing by Kathy Keller

First Edition   2009

ISBN 978-0-918860-64-4

Contents

Preface

It's a most challenging time to be alive. Health-care costs are on the rise. Medications proliferate both in number and in strength. Yet, more people are falling victim to degenerative diseases. Our environment is becoming more polluted as pesticides and other chemicals enter lakes, rivers, and our drinking water. More people means more automobiles, more factories, and more pollutants released into the air we breathe.

Most people believe there is no way out but to accept what the doctor says and what fate has in store. A growing number of people, however, are discovering a different way. While control of our external environment is more difficult, control of our internal environment is each person's responsibility. We determine what we eat, drink, feel, think, and believe each day. What we choose leads us toward health or toward illness.

This book provides information on how dietary and lifestyle choices affect acid and alkaline balance in particular and over all health in general. The more we learn, the more we practice, and the more we believe that changing any condition is possible, the less likely we are to become victims blindly following the advice of others. We become free individuals who can think for ourselves.

The book begins with a simplified overview of acid-and-alkaline theory in Chapter 1. While it is not necessary to completely understand the chemistry, the conclusion that eating a daily diet that contains more alkaline-forming foods than acid-forming ones is most important. There are many ways to determine excess acidity and these methods are detailed in Chapter 2.

The major focus of this book is on the acid-forming or alkaline-forming effects of foods. Chapter 3 contains the acid-forming or alkaline-forming effect of foods within each of the major food groups. There is also a listing (Chapter 5) of most foods in alphabetical order. Lifestyle factors influence the acid-forming and alkaline-forming effects in one direction or the other as presented in Chapter 4.

Herman Aihara first published his thoughts on acid and alkaline in 1971 and his 1986 revised edition of *Acid and Alkaline* started the current interest in acid-and-alkaline theory. I worked with Herman from 1978 to 1998 when he passed away and am very happy that this companion to his work is now completed. Acid and alkaline is an evolving field and I encourage everyone to see the conclusion (Chapter 6) for resources for further study.

Each of us knows what's best for us. The more we know about subjects like acid and alkaline the better we can evaluate what doctors, family, friends, and others advise. This book is useful for people in perfect health, for people with minor complaints, for people with any illness, and for people with a life-threatening disease. May all find here the inspiration to become healthy, happy, and free.

– Carl Ferré
April, 2009

Chapter 1

Overview of Acid and Alkaline

Our health is directly related to the condition of our internal bodily fluids. The condition of our internal bodily fluids is directly influenced by the foods we eat and by our daily activities. While there are many other factors involved in over all health, the study of acid and alkaline can be particularly advantageous. This book provides a basic understanding of acid and alkaline and ways it can be used for improved health.

Chemistry Simplified

The chemistry of acid and alkaline is quite complex and can be overwhelming. Here is a simplified explanation. Every substance is made up of many atoms. Each atom has a nucleus containing positively charged protons and negatively charged electrons in orbit around the nucleus. If the amount of positive charges and negative charges are equal the atom is stable (or inactive). As atoms come into contact with other atoms, an electron may be lost or gained through a process called "ionization." Ionization upsets the neutral state and makes the atom chemically unstable (or active).

No living thing can live without water. Chemically, a water molecule is two hydrogen atoms and one oxygen atom (H_2O). In it's neutral state, hydrogen contains one proton and one electron. If the electron is lost, the result in water is a hydroxonium ion (H_3O^+). It has an extra proton, a positive charge, and is a proton donor. Such an ion is looking for an electron in order to balance its chemical

pH Values of Body Fluids
from acid to alkaline

Stomach juice	1.7-2.0
Urine	4.5-8.0 (varies greatly)
Skin (outer layers)	around 5.5
Small Intestines	around 6.0
Saliva (healthy)	6.5-7.4 (varies greatly)
Skin (inner layers)	around 7.2
Blood	7.35-7.45
Pancreatic Juice	7.5-8.8
Large Intestines	around 8.0

charge. If an electron is gained, the result in water is a hydroxyl ion (OH⁻). This ion has a negative charge and is a proton acceptor. Such an ion has an extra electron, a negative charge, and is looking for an ion with an electron shortage to balance its chemical charge.

Every substance is made up of many atoms—some in an inactive neutral state, others that are positively charged (or proton donors), and others that are negatively charged (or proton acceptors). If the proton donors and proton acceptors are exactly equal, the substance is neutral. If there is an excess of proton donors, the substance is an acid. If there is an excess of proton acceptors, the substance is an alkaline.

The pH Scale

Scientists developed a way to determine the relative strength of any substance—the pH scale. The pH scale is based on the activity of hydrogen in a solution. The pH scale relates directly to the number of hydroxonium ions (H_3O^+) and the number of hydroxyl ions (OH⁻) in distilled water at 25 degrees C. Because there is one gram of each in every 10,000,000 liters of pure water ($1/10^7$ or 10^{-7}), a neutral pH is assigned the value of 7.0.

If there are more hydroxonium ions, the pH value goes down

(below 7.0) and the substance is an acid. Hydroxonium ions lack electrons and are looking for electrons to "consume" from other substances. If there are more hydroxyl ions the pH value goes up (above 7.0) and the substance is an alkaline. Hydroxyl ions have excess electrons and "donate" them to other substances.

It is important to understand the relative strength indicated by the pH values. A substance with ten grams of hydroxonium ions and one gram of hydroxyl ions in 10,000,000 liters has a pH value is 6.0 (10/107 or 1/106 or 10-6). Such a substance, although only a 1.0 difference on the pH scale, is 10 times more acid. Thus, a pH value of 5.0 is 10 times more acid than a pH of 6.0 and 100 times more acid than a pH of 7.0. A pH value of 4.0 is 1,000 times more acid than a pH of 7.0. A pH value of 3.0 is 10,000 times more acid than a pH of 7.0. A pH value of 2.0 is 100,000 times more acid than a pH of 7.0.

Every substance can be measured and assigned a pH value. Because the pH scale is logarithmic, pH values can go below zero. The most acidic substances found in nature are around -5.0—a trillion times more acid than a pH value of 7.0. The most alkaline substances found in nature are around 14.0—ten thousand times more alkaline than a pH value of 7.0.

Acid-Forming Versus Alkaline-Forming Foods

Foods contain both acids and alkalines and an overall pH value for each one can be determined. A typical meal contains some foods that are more acid and some foods that are more alkaline.

Foods that are more alkaline have an alkalinizing effect on the body. This effect is often referred to as "alkaline forming." However, foods that are more acid may have either an acidifying effect or an alkalinizing effect. Acid foods that have an acidifying effect are called "acid forming" while acid foods that have an alkalinizing effect are called "alkaline forming." A brief look at acid foods reveals the reason why an acid food can produce an alkaline-forming effect when metabolized.

There are two types of acids—strong (or fixed) acids and weak (or volatile) acids. Strong acids such as uric acid, sulfuric acid, and phosphoric acid are fairly stable and resist combining. The liver and the kidneys work hard to eliminate them and, because the kidneys can process only a fixed amount each day, any excess is stored in the body. Animal proteins are the main source of strong acids.

Weak acids such as citric acid and oxalic acid combine more easily and are processed and eliminated mostly by the lungs. To eliminate more of these acids, we simply breathe faster and/or more deeply. Vegetal foods contain mostly weak acids. Because these weak acids are eliminated through the lungs, the net result on the body is most often alkaline forming and not acid forming. Here is a brief explanation of this process.

When we eat any food it enters the stomach. The pH value of the stomach is around 2.0—100,000 times more acid than a pH value of 7.0. All foods become acidic in this environment. This acidic environment is necessary for our survival as it allows foods to be broken down so that nutrients can be absorbed into the body. Because all foods become acidic in the stomach, some people think a study of acid and alkaline is not important. This author and many other researchers disagree.

What remains of the food ("ash") next goes into the small intestines where a typical pH value is around 6.0. This transformation occurs as bile with an alkaline pH of 7.8 to 8.2 enters from the gall bladder and pancreatic juice with an alkaline pH of 7.5 to 8.8 enters from the pancreas. The resulting "ash" from the original food is absorbed into the body from the small intestines. Waste products go through the large intestines (pH of around 8.0) before being eliminated.

There are basically three types of "ash" that are absorbed by the small intestines. Alkaline ash from alkaline foods is used by the body to buffer acids and the over all effect is increased alkalinity. Weak acid "ash" is processed mostly by the lungs and the over all effect is either alkaline forming or acid forming depending on the amount eaten and the condition of the person eating the foods. Strong acid "ash" is processed mostly by the kidneys and the over all effect is increased acidity.

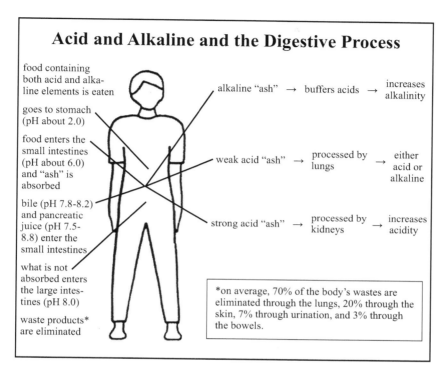

Acid and Alkaline and the Digestive Process

food containing both acid and alka- line elements is eaten

goes to stomach (pH about 2.0)

food enters the small intestines (pH about 6.0) and "ash" is absorbed

bile (pH 7.8-8.2) and pancreatic juice (pH 7.5- 8.8) enter the small intestines

what is not absorbed enters the large intes- tines (pH 8.0)

waste products* are eliminated

alkaline "ash" → buffers acids → increases alkalinity

weak acid "ash" → processed by lungs → either acid or alkaline

strong acid "ash" → processed by kidneys → increases acidity

*on average, 70% of the body's wastes are eliminated through the lungs, 20% through the skin, 7% through urination, and 3% through the bowels.

Waste products from strong acid "ash" are filtered by the kidneys and are eliminated in urine and through the skin. Skin accounts for the elimination of about 20 percent of the body's total waste products while urine accounts for about 7 percent and bowels account for 3 percent. Waste products from weak acid "ash" (and from alkaline "ash") are eliminated mostly by the lungs, which accounts for the elimination of the remaining 70 percent of the body's waste products.

Buffer System

It is so critical that the body's blood pH remain slightly alkaline at 7.35 to 7.45 that the body has elaborate buffer systems in order to accomplish this requirement. In fact, the body is so successful that what we eat has no direct effect on blood pH. It is impossible to "feel" the blood pH becoming more acid or alkaline after eating any food. Here is a brief description of the body's main buffer system.

When we eat a meal that has more alkaline-forming foods than acid-forming foods, the body is most happy. The excess alkaline is either eliminated or is stored harmlessly within the body's tissues. When we eat a meal that has more acid-forming foods than alkaline-forming foods, the body must deal with the excess acidity. If we are healthy to begin with and if this occurs infrequently, the excess acidity is handled by the lungs and kidneys.

Overeating acid-forming foods over a long time is a problem. As we more frequently eat meals that are more acid forming, problems begin to emerge. There is a limit to how much acid the lungs and kidneys can eliminate. When we overload the system, the excess acids must be buffered. After any excess alkalinity is used, alkaline substances are "borrowed" from the tissues of non-vital internal organs.

The process is really quite simple. We benefit when our internal environment is slightly alkaline. We experience problems when our internal environment becomes too acidic. The more acidic our internal environment the more troublesome the disorders we face. And, all disorders—no matter what the cause—thrive in an acidic environment. Still, both acid-forming and alkaline-forming foods are required for a healthy condition—becoming too alkaline, although rare, also can be detrimental.

It makes perfect sense to eat a daily diet that contains more alkaline-forming foods than acid-forming ones. This book provides the information for such a diet. The cost is minimal when compared with the high cost of "health" care and medications, most of which are highly acid forming by the way. We all make choices in our daily lives. Some decisions lead us toward sickness and sadness. Other decisions lead us toward health and happiness. The choice is ours.

Chapter 2

How to Tell Your Condition

Ways to determine acidity and alkalinity in the body range from analysis of one's health changes to elaborate tests that analyze every bodily fluid. The methods used or required depend on each person's current situation. People who discover acid and alkaline while still relatively healthy have more time for study and analysis than those who are already dealing with a life-threatening illness. Still, everyone, regardless of condition, can benefit from the information in this book.

Understanding the basis of acid and alkaline is simple. Preliminary analysis can be done at home. This book provides definable values for foods and activities. The solution for anyone with a minor imbalance is easy—eat slightly more alkaline-forming foods at every meal. Anyone with a major imbalance may need to increase the proportion of alkaline-forming foods, study additional literature, or consult with a health care professional.

Health Change Analysis

Most of us can remember a time when we were truly healthy. We woke up refreshed and ready to meet the challenges of the day—and we greeted each new day with gratitude and enthusiasm. We also can remember a time when we literally had to drag ourselves out of bed. We were fatigued all day or got sick often. Analyzing past and current health and energy levels can be most revealing.

Start by making a list of every cold, flu, other disease, or period of fatigue you've experienced in the past 10 years. Include when it began, medications, or other action taken, and when it ended if it has. Be as thorough and as honest as you can. Consider changes in your health since childhood. Do you have the same energy levels and enthusiasm? Have there been changes in your physical, mental, or spiritual health and outlook on life? Have these changes improved your life?

Initial signals

Negative changes in health are our body's way of warning us that changes in diet and lifestyle are needed. Athough all changes in health may have multiple causes, initial signals usually indicate that a change in diet and lifestyle is required. Ridding the body of excess acidity is easy and relatively inexpensive—simply eat more alkaline-forming than acid-forming foods on a daily basis. This action alone will begin the journey toward recovery and better health. Following is a list of changes in health that may indicate excess acidity. Be sure to use the other methods in this chapter to confirm.

Activity reduced due to being "too tired" or abnormally active (hyperactivity)

Allergies to food and greater sensitivity to airborne particles such as cut grass

Bladder, urethra, or rectal irritation, or burning sensation

Breath, rapid panting without much exertion

Chemical sensitivities to odors such as gas heaters or pilot lights

Circulation poor, frequently feel cold or chilled, especially hands and feet

Coughs and sore throats, respiratory tract more sensitive to cold

Dizziness, increased or more frequent

Energy, lowered, harder to get up in the morning and/or tire more easily

Exercise, greater difficulty recovering strength after exertion

Enthusiasm for life diminished

Eyes more sensitive to smoke and other irritants and tear more easily

Face, very pale showing signs of anemia

Fatigue, frequent or constant

Feelings of an inability to cope, increased or more frequent

Gums more sensitive or inflamed

Hair, split ends and a lot falls out at one time

Headaches, mild and/or recurring

Heartbeat, rapid or irregular

Infections more frequent

Joints creak, such as when rotating the shoulders

Lips, cracked, especially at the corners

Mental awareness, dulled or increasing loss of concentration

Mouth, metallic taste or acidic all the time

Nails, split or break more easily or have "white" spots on them

Neck, stiff or tight

Nose, frequently runs, contains excess mucous, or feels stuffy

Pain, muscular or joint pains that move around the body or greater sensitivity to pain

Panic attacks, increased nervousness or agitation over "little" things (fear or anxiety)

Pre-menstrual syndrome (PMS)—pre-menstrual and menstrual cramping

Sex drive, reduced or lacking

Skin, overly acidic leading to pimples and/or acne

Skin problems, such as overly dry, red, swollen, irritated, itching, and/or splits and cracks

Stressed out more easily or greater difficulty dealing with stress—increased irritability

Stomach acid excessive causing acid indigestion, nausea, acid reflux, bloating, or heartburn

Stools, discolored or loose leading to diarrhea

Stools, increasingly hard, leading to constipation, slow peristaltic movement

Teeth, loose and/or more sensitive to hot or cold foods or drinks

Thoughts, more sad or depressing

Tongue, white coating

Urine, acidic, strong smelling, hot (burning sensation)
Urination, more frequent
Vision, hearing, smelling, tasting changes

Named disorders

Most of us think these signals are part of the aging process. We take over-the-counter medications to relieve the symptoms without concern for understanding and/or curing the underlying cause. The result is a named disorder that often requires a prescription. This action might relieve the symptoms, but, if the underlying cause is not cured, the result is greater problems. Following is a list of changes in health that may indicate excess acidity. Be sure to use the other methods in this chapter to confirm.

Bones: fractures are slow to heal, osteomyelitis, osteoporosis, rickets

Circulation: anemia, atherosclerosis, cardiovascular disease, hypoglycemia or low blood sugar, internal bleeding, leg cramps or spasms, low blood pressure,

Eyes, nose, and ears: cataracts, conjunctivitis, coronary occlusion, earaches, glaucoma, macular degeneration, sinusitis

General: alcoholism, anal fistula, obesity

Glands: hyperthyroidism, hypothyroidism

Immune system: immune system depression

Infections, fungal: athletes' foot, Candida albicans, Celiac disease, vaginitis

Infections, bacterial: staph or strep, urinary tract

Infections, viral: colds and flu

Intestines: appendicitis, colitis, enteritis, ileitis, intestinal cramps

Joints and tendons: arthritis, bursitis, fibromyalgia, gout, joint hyperlaxity, numbness and tingling, rheumatism, osteoarthritis, tendonitis

Kidneys/bladder: kidney or bladder stones, nephritis, toxemia

Liver/gall bladder: cirrhosis, cystitis, gallstones, urethritis

Lungs/respiration: asthma, bronchitis, emphysema, hay fever, pneumonia

Mental and head: depression, hallucinations, migraine headaches, obsessive-compulsive disorder, memory loss, insomnia, stuttering

Nerves and nervous system: epilepsy, neuritis (nerve pain, tenacious or migrant), sciatica

Sexual: cystic breasts, endometriosis, fibroid uterine tumors, heavy periods, impotence, infertility, miscarriages, prostate enlargement, prostatitis, utero or vulva inflammation, vaginal discharge

Skin: eczema, hives, Herpes I or II, psoriasis

Spine: herniated disks, locking vertebrae, slipped vertebrae

Stomach: abdominal pain, gastritis, ulcers (stomach or duodenal)

Teeth and gums: dental cavities, gingivitis, gum disease, mouth ulcers, tooth nerve pain

Throat: adenoids, angina, enlarged tonsils, laryngitis

Serious or systemic diseases

Most of us go to the doctor once any of these symptoms or disorders advances beyond our ability to cope with them. We get a prescription and take medication, which may or may not work. The medication may relieve the symptoms but most often does nothing to heal the underlying cause. We fall victim to a more serious or systemic disease. Following is a list of changes in health that may indicate excess acidity. Be sure to use the other methods in this chapter to confirm.

Alzheimer's disease
Bleeding ulcers
Cancer, all forms
Crohn's disease
Diabetes, type I or II
Down's syndrome

Heart attacks
Hodgkin's disease
Leukemia
Multiple sclerosis
Myasthenia gravis
Parkinson's disease
Rheumatoid arthritis
Sarcoidosis
Schizophrenia
Scleroderma
Strokes
Systemic lupus erythematosis
Tuberculosis

All these indicators, disorders, and serious diseases thrive in an acidic environment. We have some control over the health of our internal environment by the foods and drinks we consume and by our daily activities. We are not victims. If we are in good health, we can maintain it. If we experience any of the initial indicators of health changes, we can take steps to return to good health. If we already have a disorder at any level of progression, we can help remedy it by providing the best internal environment possible—one that is slightly alkaline and not overly acidic.

Diet and Lifestyle Analysis

An analysis of daily diet and lifestyle can be helpful both in determining the cause of one's present condition and as a way to maintain a good one or to change a bad one.

Start by writing down all the foods and drinks consumed at each meal and during the day for a period of one week. Determine if this list is typical of your daily diet. Include times you eat out at restaurants or with friends, especially if you do this often.

Look up the foods on your list in the charts found in books on acid and alkaline, online, or in future installments of this series. Write down the acid-forming or alkaline-forming value for each one.

Note that if you have any named disorder or more serious disease, move the value in the acid-forming direction. All disorders not only thrive in an acidic environment but also compromise the body's ability to process acid-forming foods. Also, move the value in the acidic direction if you ate on the run or in a chaotic environment. Add up the values for each meal and snacks. Notice if the diet includes more acid-forming foods or more alkaline-forming foods. This process should give a picture of whether or not your diet is more acidic or more on the alkaline side.

Lifestyle factors need to be evaluated as well. The effect of various activities and stress levels can be found in Chapter 4 beginning on page 57. A quick glance shows that many of our daily activities are acid forming. The more acid-forming factors in our daily life, the more the diet needs to be adjusted to the alkaline side. An appropriate diet for a monk who is meditating most of the day is different from someone who commutes to work in heavy traffic and works all day at a stressful job.

Urinary and Saliva Analysis

The acidity or alkalinity of any liquid can be measured by the use of hydrion (litmus) paper. This paper turns red when it comes into contact with an acidic solution and blue when it comes into contact with an alkaline solution. The strength of the color is matched to a chart for an approximate pH value. Anyone who has a swimming pool and has tested the pH of the water is familiar with this process. Hydrion or litmus paper can be purchased from pharmacies or drugstores.

The advantage of hydrion paper is that it is easy to use. The main disadvantages are that the results are easy to misinterpret and that it can not be used for measuring the internal fluids. An acidic result when testing the urine may simply mean the body is doing what it's supposed to do—getting rid of acid wastes. The pH of saliva varies greatly and is only indicative of the pH of the saliva at the moment of the test—it does not mean the internal fluids are the same value, or even anywhere close.

Many years ago research scientist Jym Moon attended the French Meadows Camp—an annual macrobiotic summer camp founded by Herman Aihara, author of *Acid and Alkaline*. This scientist brought litmus paper to test people's saliva. He measured his saliva at the beginning of his lecture to demonstrate how easy a test it was. The pH of his saliva measured a neutral 7.0. He gave an enlightening talk on the scientific aspects of acid and alkaline. After two hours of lecturing and answering questions, he measured his saliva again. This time, the paper turned red and measured 5.0. Without any food or drink, his saliva had changed from 7.0 to 5.0 over the course of two hours.

"According to this I should be dead!" he exclaimed giving a wide grin. He then explained that lecturing or any other stressful activity is acid forming. A change in the pH of his saliva did not mean that his internal fluids had changed at all. Measuring saliva pH is not that beneficial without proper understanding.

To use saliva pH in a beneficial way, measure it the first thing after getting up in the morning before putting anything in your mouth. Rinse your mouth with your own saliva while rubbing your teeth with your tongue and spit this out. Next, spit some saliva into a clean spoon and place the hydrion paper in it for one or two seconds following the directions on the package. Record the reading. Do this for one week or longer and look for changes. Evaluate any changes based on what you ate and what you did the day before.

Measuring urinary pH can be more revealing and should be done to confirm saliva pH readings. Each urination of the day can be measured, recorded, and evaluated. When measuring urinary pH, either urinate directly into a container or onto the paper for 1 to 2 seconds. Measure or collect urine during the middle of your urination. Record the first urination and the readings from each urination before meals or at least 1 hour after meals. Do this for one week or longer noting any changes in diet or lifestyle from your normal routine.

Analysis of the results is fairly simple but can be misleading if done without the other methods of analysis in this chapter. We all have acidic wastes that must be eliminated. The first urination of the day should be acidic because it contains acidic wastes that the kidneys have processed and accumulated during the night. Check to see that your first urination of the day is less than 7.0. If it's not, most likely your body is overly acidic and accumulating acids. This acidification needs to be remedied first by eating more alkaline-forming foods than acidic-forming ones at every meal.

Look at the values for the rest of the day. Urinary pH values that are not uniform during the day indicate that the internal environment is overly acidic and needs attention. If the urinary pH is between 6.0 and 7.0 on a consistent basis, you have slight over-acidity. If the urinary pH is consistently under 6.0, the acidity is more extreme and corrections in diet and lifestyle are needed immediately. A urinary pH between 7.0 and 7.5 is a good sign as long as the first urination is acidic as discussed above.

A urinary pH above 7.5 requires additional analysis. The body attempts to rid itself of excess alkaline just as it attempts to rid itself of excess acid. Excess alkaline foods or supplements eaten or taken over a period of time can lead to a high alkaline urinary pH. Look at your dietary analysis to confirm this. Reduce the amount of alkaline supplements taken or the proportion of alkaline-to-acid-forming foods eaten so that the urinary pH falls between 7.0 and 7.5. Whole grains and beans are a good way to increase the amount of acid-forming foods for vegetarians and others not wanting to eat animal foods.

People with an acidic internal environment can have an overly high (alkaline) urinary pH. In this case, the body is having trouble processing acids in the normal way and the overload of acids causes the body to release stored alkaline substances to buffer the overload. The result is more alkaline substances eliminated through the urine. Look at your health change analysis to confirm this.

There are extremely rare cases in which glandular problems or other specific disorders cause a high urinary pH (consistently over 7.5). If changes in diet and lifestyle do not remedy the situation, medical or another health-care provider's attention is recommended.

Experimental and Intuitive Analysis

Analysis of one's health changes, diet, lifestyle, and urinary pH provides a good picture of one's over all health and the extent—if any—of acidification of the internal environment. There is another test that can be done at home if desired. This test involves intentionally eating a high acid-forming diet for 3 to 10 days followed by eating a high alkaline-forming diet for the next 3 to 10 days. Evaluate the result both in how you feel and in variations of your urinary pH readings.

People with persistent health problems related to excess acidity and urinary pH readings consistently in the acid range don't need to perform the acid-forming part of this test. If eating a high alkaline-forming diet for 3 to 10 days or longer reduces the severity of some of the initial indicators, then there is little doubt that the internal environment would benefit from a permanent change to more alkaline-forming foods then acid-forming foods at each meal. Complete recovery of these symptoms and any disorders or major diseases can take many months or years.

Most of us intuitively know what's best for us. Our internal intuitive voice speaks to us all the time. Still, we make choices that lead us away from health. We all prefer to consume the foods and drinks we enjoy. We don't want to admit that our diet may be the underlying cause of our aches and pains, illnesses, and serious disorders—yet we intuitively know it. Make a change to a high alkaline-forming diet for 10 days to 2 weeks and see for yourself.

Beyond Home Testing

Life and health include much more than acid-and-alkaline balance. What is included in this book is a simplified explanation of one of the body's important processes. If changes in acid-and-alkaline balance do not resolve troublesome changes in health, the underlying cause needs to be determined and other dietary and lifestyle changes may need to be made. Persistent and serious conditions may require further testing and help. There are many tests that can be evaluated at a medical laboratory. These tests usually require a physician's order and analysis.

The human body is a living miracle. Advances in medicine and instrumentation make greater understanding of its mechanisms and processes possible. A physician or other health-care provider who understands metabolic processes can be invaluable, especially in persistent or serious cases of acid-and-alkaline imbalance.

The number and effectiveness of alternative approaches is increasing. These include learning macrobiotic principles (yin and yang), adopting a raw foods or blood type diet, evaluating one's Ayurveda body type, and food combining to name just a few. The understanding gained from any and all approaches to health is valuable. The best guide for each of us, however, is our own body. Aches and pains that develop without a physical cause are the body's signals that changes are needed. The study of acid and alkaline (and yin and yang) helps us determine the direction of that change.

Chapter 3

Acid and Alkaline
of Foods

Many health problems from aches and pains to serious diseases are the body's attempt to clean up the internal environment—eating more alkaline-forming foods than acid-forming foods at each meal is one way to help this process. Increase the proportion of alkaline-forming foods if the body's internal environment is already overly acidic. Note: It is best not to eat meals that are solely comprised of acid-forming (or alkaline-forming) foods, especially continuously for any length of time.

The acidity or alkalinity of any food is easy to determine—simply measure it with litmus paper. As we learned in Chapter 1, however, it is the effect of the food once metabolized that concerns us. Scientists have developed a method to approximate the digestive process by burning a food to ashes, adding pure water to make a solution, and then measuring its acidity or alkalinity.

Another method used to determine the likelihood of acid-forming or alkaline-forming foods involves an evaluation of the elements in the food. There are elements that are known to be acid forming and elements that are known to be alkaline forming. In theory, foods containing more acid-forming elements are acid forming and foods containing more alkaline-forming elements are more alkaline forming. The major acid-forming elements are: sulfur (S), phosphorus (P), chlorine (Cl), and iodine (I). The main alkaline-forming elements are: sodium (Na), potassium (K), calcium (Ca), magnesium (Mg), and iron (Fe).

Acid and Alkaline of Nutritional Elements

<u>Acid-forming</u>
sulfur (S)
phosphorus (P)
chlorine (Cl)
iodine (I)

<u>Alkaline-forming</u>
sodium (Na)
potassium (K)
calcium (Ca)
magnesium (Mg)
iron (Fe)

The calcium (alkaline-forming element) to phosphorous (acid-forming element) ratio is used in a similar way to help determine whether a food is acid forming or alkaline forming. All of these methods, however, are only approximations of what actually happens within the body.

The final method used to determine acid-forming and alkaline-forming foods is personal experience. Researchers evaluate the effects of foods on themselves and on their clients and then move foods in the acid-forming or alkaline-forming direction. Each of us is unique and reacts to foods and activities in different ways. Any values for foods or activities in this book—or in any book for that matter—are to be used only as general guidelines. Some foods are listed as alkaline forming by one researcher and acid forming by another. Tests done in a laboratory or analysis of acid-forming elements and alkaline-forming elements in foods can only approximate what happens in the body. Some authors add their own experience to the mix. And, because each person's internal environment is different, the values are approximate in every chart in every book.

What is important for each of us is what happens in our own body. Daily monitoring is most beneficial. A food that is acid forming, while the internal environment is overly acidic, may become alkaline forming once the excess acidity is neutralized. For this reason, people who have trouble processing acids may need to limit or avoid acidic foods until this condition improves even though the foods are listed as being alkaline forming in the body. These acidic foods are placed in italics in the food charts that follow in Chapter 5.

The food charts in this book contain a comparative value from C9 (severely acid forming) to K9 (extremely alkaline forming) followed by a range of values within which the food usually falls. There are many factors—as will be pointed out—that move a food in the acid-forming or alkaline-forming direction. Here is a list of the comparative values and an explanation of what each means:

C9: severely acid forming
C8: exceedingly acid forming
C7: strongly acid forming
C6: highly acid forming
C5: moderately acid forming
C4: generally acid forming
C3: fairly acid forming
C2: mildly acid forming
C1: slightly acid forming
C0: imperceptibly acid forming
K0: imperceptibly alkaline forming
K1: slightly alkaline forming
K2: mildly alkaline forming
K3: fairly alkaline forming
K4: generally alkaline forming
K5: moderately alkaline forming
K6: highly alkaline forming
K7: strongly alkaline forming
K8: exceedingly alkaline forming
K9: extremely alkaline forming

Foods in General

Foods can be classified in general as acid forming or alkaline forming by their protein, fat, carbohydrate, and mineral composition. Foods that are high in protein, fat, and carbohydrates are acid forming while foods that are high in vitamins and minerals are alkaline forming. The chart on page 28 lists the general acid-forming or alkaline-forming effect of various food groups. A complete listing of most foods can be found beginning on page 66.

This chart clearly shows the difficulty in neutralizing the acid-forming effect of a meat-and-sugar diet. We are encouraged to eat more fruits and vegetables. This approach is fine as long as the body isn't already overloaded with acidity. In this case, fruits are acid forming and not alkaline forming—they contribute to the problem. It is difficult to eat enough vegetables to counter the quantities of meat and sugar many people consume.

Salt contains sodium—an alkaline-forming element—and eating more of it would appear to be a solution. However, because meat is also high in fat and excess sugar turns to fat in the body, we are encouraged to limit our salt (sodium) intake because the combination leads to high blood pressure and other heart-related problems. No wonder health-care costs are on the rise!

Some people turn to more grains and beans as protein and fat sources. This approach can work as long as enough protein and fat is included in the diet, enough vegetables are eaten, and refined sugar is limited or eliminated completely. Fruits are alkaline forming once the body is not overloaded with acidity and once we have no trouble processing the acids they contain.

One of the first steps toward a healthier and happier life is ridding our internal environment of excess acidity or—in a few rare cases—excess alkalinity. One of the objectives of this book is to provide information on how to eat the foods we enjoy in a more balanced and healthy way. Another objective is to introduce a great variety of foods that are unfamiliar to most people. An excellent cookbook for preparing whole grains, beans, and vegetables is Julia Ferré's *Basic Macrobiotic Cooking, Twentieth Anniversary Edition*

Acid and Alkaline of Food Groups

	Alkaline ← + neutral – → Acid
	k9 k8 k7 k6 k5 k4 k3 k2 k1 kc0 c1 c2 c3 c4 c5 c6 c7 c8 c9
Grains,whole	---+---------X--------
Grains, refined	-----------X--------
Sprouts from grains and beans	----------X--------
Beans, fresh	-----X------
Beans, dried	-------X--------
Vegetables	---------X----------
Sea vegetables	------X------
Pickles, naturally made with sea salt	----X---------------
Pickles, commercial	-----X -----
Fruits (depends on ability to process)*	------------X-----------------------------------
Nuts and seeds	----------X----------
Herbs and spices	---------X---------
Vegetable oils	----------X----------------------
Salt, sea	-------X-------
Salt, refined table	-----X-----
Fish (lean is less acid forming)	----------X----------
Eggs	--------X--------
Poultry	----------X-------
Dairy products	------------X-----------
Red meats	-------X------
Water (depends on composition)	---------X------------
Alcohol (natural is less acid forming)	-------------X-------
Beverages, sugared	
Sugar (refined)	----X---
Sweenteners (artifical)	--X--
Drugs and medications (most)	-x-

The "x" indicates the over all average of the food group and the dashed line indicates the average range of each food group.

* Fruits and other foods that have a large amount of acids can be more difficult to process, especially for people whose health is compromised in any way. Such people will find that these foods are acid forming for them while alkaline forming for others. See the section on fruit, page 37-41.

(G.O.M.F. 2007). Here is a more detailed look at each of the food groups.

Whole Grains

Whole grains are becoming more and more popular as the main component of daily meals. Whole grains contain all major nutrient groups needed by the body: carbohydrates, protein, fat, vitamins, minerals, and fiber. The composition and percentage of each nutrient group make each whole grain either more acid forming or more alkaline forming. Amaranth (a relative of spinach), buckwheat (a relative of rhubarb), and quinoa (goosefoot family) are not part of the grass family but are used primarily as grains and are listed here with the whole grains.

Millet contains a fair amount of silica, which is an acid-forming element. Individuals who have trouble processing silica will find millet to be acid forming and may need to avoid eating millet until his or her internal condition improves. Persons who do not have trouble processing silica will find millet to be alkaline forming and a good food for restoring minerals to the body.

A similar effect can occur with any food that an individual has trouble digesting—some people are allergic to wheat for example. People allergic to a certain food—a possible sign of excess acidity—will find the effect of that food to be more acidic because of the added stress required to process it.

Here is a list of factors that affect acid and alkaline effect: "+" indicates an alkaline-forming direction, while "–" indicates an acid-forming direction.

1. Move +3 to +4 for whole grains that are acid forming provided each mouthful of grain is chewed 100 times or more. For example, brown rice is listed as c4. If each mouthful is chewed 100 times or more move its value to c1 or c0. There is much less effect, if any, on grains that are already alkaline forming. The effect only works with grains and is due to the action of the enzyme ptyalin in the saliva. This enzyme action is greatly diminished if vegetables, fruit, or other foods are in the mouth at the same time as the grain.

Acid and Alkaline of Grains

	Alkaline ← + neutral − → Acid k9 k8 k7 k6 k5 k4 k3 k2 k1 kc0 c1 c2 c3 c4 c5 c6 c7 c8 c9
Amaranth	----X---------
Barley, whole grain	------X------
Brown basmati rice	----X----
Brown rice	------X-----
Buckwheat groats	----------------X----
Bulgur (cracked wheat)	--------X---
Corn, blue	-X-------
Corn, whole (yellow or white, maize)	------X------
Couscous, white flour	----X----
Couscous, whole wheat flour	----X---
Flour, white wheat	----X---
Flour, whole wheat	----X----
Japonica rice	-X-------
Millet	---X-----------------------------
Oats, rolled (oatmeal), unsweetened	--------------------X----
Oats, whole	------------------X-------
Pastas, from white flour	----X----
Pastas, from whole grains	------X------
Quinoa	----X---------
Rye, whole grain	------X------
Sprouts: amaranth, millet, or quinoa	-------X----
Sprouts, from other grains	----X----
Sweet brown rice	----X----
Tef	-X--------
White bread, yeasted	----X---
Whole wheat	----X----
Whole wheat bread	----X---
Wild rice	----X---

The "x" indicates the over all average of the food and the dashed line indicates the average range of each food. Foods in italics contain a large amount of acid and are acid forming for some people and alkaline forming for others, see pages 37 and 41.

Thoroughly chewing one's food is valuable for many other reasons and is highly recommended.

2. Move +1 to +2 if the grain is cooked with sea salt. Note: refined table salt is acid forming and is not recommended—if used, move −1 to −2.

3. Move −1 to −2 if grains are refined. Most refined grains are listed in the complete food tables beginning on page 66. Note: discard refined grains if they have become rancid or have a harsh after taste.

4. Move −1 to −2 if whole grains are used to make bread or other flour-based products. Toasting bread reduces its acid-forming effect by the way.

5. Move −1 to −3 if sugar is added to the grain.

6. Move −1 to −3 if hard-kernelled grains are not soaked for 4 to 8 hours or dry roasted prior to cooking. Dried grains contain enzyme inhibitors that interfere with digestion. Soaking or dry roasting the whole grain before cooking neutralizes this effect.

The study and use of whole grains can be very beneficial. Amaranth is higher in protein and calcium than milk and is good for weight gain. Buckwheat contains all eight essential amino acids and helps neutralize acidic wastes in the body. Oats are high in sodium and unsaturated fat and help improve one's resistance to stress. Quinoa is high in iron, is equal to milk in protein quality, and has more calcium than milk. Tef is high in protein and is a rich source of calcium, iron, zinc, and copper. Full information on each of the whole grains and grain products in this book is available in *The New Whole Foods Encyclopedia* by Rebecca Wood.

Vegetables

Vegetables are an integral part of any well-rounded diet. They are most all alkaline forming and are essential for neutralizing the acid-forming effects of proteins, fats, and carbohydrates. Tomatoes are a fruit and peas, green beans, and lima beans are legumes. Tomatoes and green beans are included in the following chart of selected vegetables because they are used like vegetables.

These listings are for fresh organic vegetables. The way a vegetable is grown, harvested, and processed moves its acid-forming or

Acid and Alkaline of Vegetables

	Alkaline ← + neutral − → Acid k9 k8 k7 k6 k5 k4 k3 k2 k1 kc0 c1 c2 c3 c4 c5 c6 c7 c8 c9
Broccoli	-------X----------
Cabbage	----------X-------
Carrots, commercial (canned)	----------------X------
Carrots, organic	-------X-------
Cauliflower	----X-------
Celery	---------X--------
Cucumbers	----------X-------
Green beans	----------X-----
Kale	----------X--------
Leeks	----X----
Lettuce, iceberg	----X----
Mustard greens	---------X--------
Onions	--------------X-------
Parsnips	--------------X-------
Peas, fresh green	---------X-------------------
Potatoes, with peel	------X----------
Potatoes, without skins	--X------------------
Radishes	----------X----------
Salad greens, mixed	----X----
Scallions (green onions)	----X-------
Sea vegetables, most	----X-------
Shiitake mushrooms	-------X----
Summer squash: crookneck, zucchini	----X----
Sweet corn (corn on the cob)	----X-------
Sweet potatoes	-------X---
Tomatoes	----------X---------------
Turnips	-------X-------
Winter squash, most	---------X----

The "x" indicates the over all average of the food and the dashed line indicates the average range of each food. Foods in italics contain a large amount of acid and are acid forming for some people and alkaline forming for others, see pages 37 and 41.

alkaline-forming effect one direction or the other. Here is a list of factors that move vegetables in an acid-forming direction.

1. Move –1 to –2 if vegetables have been pre-cooked, frozen, canned, or non-organic.
2. Move –2 to –4 if vegetables are grown with chemicals, are processed with preservatives, or are sugared. The acid-forming effect of these actions should not be overlooked or underestimated.
3. Move –1 to –2 if acid-forming dressings are added to vegetables or salads.
4. Move –1 to –2 if vegetables are boiled and the cooking water is discarded. Some of the minerals that make vegetables alkaline forming are in the cooking water—use in soups to return this benefit.
5. Move –1 if vegetables are over cooked.
6. Move –1 to –3 if edible skins are discarded. For example, most of the nutrients of a potato are found just under the skin—alkaline-forming minerals are discarded along with skin.

The fresher and sweeter vegetables taste and the sooner they are eaten after harvesting, the more alkaline forming the effect. The study and use of a great variety of vegetables can be very beneficial. There are many families and each contains useful vegetables that are relatively unknown.

One vegetable family deserves special consideration. Vegetables grown in the sea are high in minerals and are among the most alkaline-forming foods found in nature. Sea vegetables (or sea weeds) are used in many processed foods—even ice cream. Most of us have a lot of seaweeds in our lives without even knowing it. Information on how to prepare vegetables and sea vegetables can be found in *Basic Macrobiotic Cooking: Twentieth Anniversary Edition* by Julia Ferré. Full information on each of the vegetables and sea vegetables listed in this book is available in *The New Whole Foods Encyclopedia* by Rebecca Wood.

Acid and Alkaline of Pickles and Condiments

	Alkaline ← + neutral – → Acid k9 k8 k7 k6 k5 k4 k3 k2 k1 kc0 c1 c2 c3 c4 c5 c6 c7 c8 c9
Bran pickles, nuka	----x----
Brine pickles	----x----
Daikon pickles (takuwan)	----x----
Dill pickles, homemade with apple cider vinegar	----x----
Dill pickles, homemade with sea salt	----x----
Miso pickles	----x----
Sake pickles	-x-------
Salt pickles, using sea salt	----x----
Soy sauce pickles	----x----
Umeboshi pickles	---x----
Arrowroot powder	----x----
Barley miso	--------------x-------
Brown rice vinegar, traditionally brewed	----x----
Gomashio (sesame salt)	----x----
Kudzu root	----x----
Mayonnaise, natural, homemade	----x----
Miso, most kinds	--------------x-------
Mustard, natural, stone-ground	------------------x----
Salt, iodized table	----x----
Salt, sea	----x--------------------
Salt, table, refined	------------------------------x-------
Soy sauce	----x---------------
Soy sauce, with sugar and additives	---x-------------
Sweet brown rice vinegar	----x----
Umeboshi paste	----x----
Umeboshi vinegar	----x------------
White vinegar	-------x----

The "x" indicates the over all average of the food and the dashed line indicates the average range of each food.

Pickles

Pickles are vegetables that have been preserved in brine, vinegar, or other marinade. Naturally processed pickles are extremely alkaline forming and are very useful for helping neutralize excess acidity. Pickles are eaten with a meal, at the end of a meal as a digestive aid, or as a snack between meals. A chart of pickles and condiments, and their general alkaline-forming and acid-forming effects, is on the preceding page.

The alkaline-forming or acid-forming effect of pickles depends mostly on the solution in which the vegetables are preserved. The effect of this solution is so strong that the quality of the original vegetable influences the final product much less than if eaten without pickling. Here is a list of factors that move pickles in an acid-forming ("–") direction.

1. Move –2 to –4 if refined salt is used in pickles rather than sea salt.
2. Move –1 to –2 if vegetables used to make pickles were grown with chemicals or processed with preservatives or sugar.
3. Move –2 to –3 if chemical additives or sugar are added at any time during processing.

Condiments and Herbs and Spices

Condiments and herbs and spices can be very useful to help neutralize excess acidity because most are alkaline forming. These foods and products add special flavor to food. They may be used in cooking or may be added at the table when eating. A chart of common herbs and spices and their general alkaline-forming and acid-forming effects is on the following page.

These listings are for products without added sugar unless indicated. The way each food or product is grown, harvested, and processed moves the alkaline-forming or acid-forming effect one direction or the other. Here is a list of factors that move herbs and spices in an acid-forming direction.

1. Move –1 to –2 if herbs or spices are pre-ground or old. Oils deteriorate after grinding.

Acid and Alkaline of Herbs and Spices

	Alkaline ← + neutral – → Acid k9 k8 k7 k6 k5 k4 k3 k2 k1 kc0 c1 c2 c3 c4 c5 c6 c7 c8 c9
Anise	----X----
Basil	----X-------
Bay leaf	----X-------
Black pepper	----X----
Cayenne pepper (capsicum)	-------X--------------
Chamomile	----X----
Chili pepper	----X----
Cinnamon	----X-----------
Citrus peel (zest)	----X----
Cloves	----X----
Coriander leaf (cilantro)	----X----
Coriander seeds	----X----
Curry powder	-X------------
Garlic	-------X--------------
Ginger, powdered	----X----
Ginger root, fresh	----X--------
Herbs, leafy green	----X-------
Mint	----X----
Nutmeg	----X-----------
Oregano	----X-------
Paprika	----------X------------
Rosemary	----X----
Sage	----X----
Spices, in general	------------------X--------
Tarragon	----X----
Thyme	-------X----
Turmeric	----X----
Vanilla extract	--------X--------

The "x" indicates the over all average of the food and the dashed line indicates the average range of each food.

2. Move −1 to −2 if herbs and spices are imported and have been sterilized. Fumigation is required for herbs and spices entering the United States and this process degrades the alkaloids in some plants.
3. Move −2 to −4 if herbs and spices or products used to make condiments are grown with chemicals, are processed with preservatives, or are sugared.

The more pleasing the aroma and the greater the vibrancy of condiments, herbs, and spices, the better, and the more alkaline forming they are. People who are avoiding or reducing meat and sugar intake benefit greatly from the study and use of naturally made condiments and high quality herbs and spices. They can turn an otherwise bland diet into one that is flavorful, enjoyable, and healthful.

Fruits

Fruits freshly picked off the tree or vine and eaten on a hot summer day are delicious and satisfying. They provide vitamins and minerals and a quick burst of energy from the sugars they contain. Most fruits also contain a lot of acids and for this reason may be alkaline forming or acid forming in effect. A chart of selected freshly picked, sun-ripened organic fruits and their general alkaline-forming and acid-forming effects is on page 38.

There is more confusion about the alkaline-forming or acid-forming effect of fruits than any other food group. Fruits contain a great deal of weak acids, which are oxidized easily by a majority of people. Some people, however, have trouble dealing with excess acids. This trouble may be due to the person's metabolism, in general, or to the person's current health condition in particular.

People who have trouble processing foods containing a lot of acids should use the acid-forming values listed in the ranges for each fruit.

There are many factors that move fruit in a more acid-forming or alkaline-forming direction. Here is a list of factors: "+" indicates an alkaline-forming direction while "−" indicates an acid-forming direction.

Acid and Alkaline of Fruits

	Alkaline ← + neutral – → Acid
	k9 k8 k7 k6 k5 k4 k3 k2 k1 kc0 c1 c2 c3 c4 c5 c6 c7 c8 c9
Apples, sweet, unwaxed, organic	-x--------------------------------------
Applesauce, sweetened	-----------x--------
Applesauce, unsweetened	-x-----------------------------
Apricots, ripe	-x--------------------------
Apricots, unripe	-x---------------------------
Bananas	----------x-----------------
Blackberries	-------------x-----------------
Blueberries	-------x-----------------------
Cantaloupe, melons	---x-------------------------------
Cherries, sweet	-------x---------------------------
Cranberries	--------x--------------
Figs, fresh	-x--------------------------
Fruit conserves, homemade, no sugar	-x-----------------------
Fruit conserves, sugar or corn syrup	-x----
Fruits, tropical	----x---------------------------
Grapes, seedless	----x--------------------
Lemons	----x---
Olives, green	--------------x-----------------
Olives, pickled	---x-------
Oranges	---x-----------------------------------
Peaches	---x--------------------
Pears, sweet	----x------------------------------
Plums	-----------x--------------------
Raisins	--------x-----------------
Raspberries	----------------------x---------------------
Strawberries, sweet	-------------x-----------------
Umeboshi plums	----x--------
Watermelons	---x---------------------------------

The "x" indicates the over all average of the food and the dashed line indicates the average range of each food. Foods in italics contain a large amount of acid and are acid forming for some people and alkaline forming for others, see pages 37 and 41.

1. Quantity: move –1 to –2 if fruit is eaten in excess and overloads the system. Be careful with fruit juice because it is made from a large quantity of fruits and contains a great deal of acids to process.
2. Quality: move –1 to –3 if fruit is conventional (not organic) or is pre-cooked, canned, frozen, or preserved.
3. Processing: move –2 to –4 if refined sugar or chemicals are added to fruit during processing.
4. Whole food: move –1 to –3 if fruit is juiced and the pulp is discarded or if fruit is eaten whole but the edible skin is discarded.
5. Ripeness: move –1 to –2 if fruit is less ripe when picked. Fruit found in stores is often picked green and allowed to ripen in a warehouse or on the store shelf.
6. Preparation: move +1 to +2 if fruit is sliced or shredded prior to eating, allowing some oxidation to take place before eating it.
7. Cooking: move –1 to –2 the more fruit is cooked. This amount can be negated by adding sea salt when cooking.
8. Eater's condition: move –1 to –2 if you are tired, weakened, or sick when eating fruit.
9. Combination: move –1 to –2 if fruit is eaten with grain, given this combination produces excess toxic acids. Move +1 to +2 if fruit is eaten with cheese or cream as these foods have a buffering effect on foods with a great deal of weak acids.

The study and proper use of fruits can be very beneficial. Fruits that taste sour in general contain more acids than fruits that taste sweeter. The lemon is known for its sour taste and acid content yet its alkaline content is 5 times its acid content. Fruits such as plums, prunes, rhubarb, and cranberries that contain oxalic acid are more acid forming. Figs are high in calcium but have the highest sugar content of common fruits.

Care must be used when purchasing fruits that have been processed in any way. Dried fruits are a concentrated sugar source and are often sulfured (acid forming), or are otherwise altered during processing. Fruit preserves (conserves) are best when 100 percent fruit with nothing added. Most minerals are removed from fruit juice concentrate during processing leaving mostly sugar and water. It is highly acid forming and should be avoided.

Acid and Alkaline of Beans

	Alkaline ← + neutral – → Acid
	k9 k8 k7 k6 k5 k4 k3 k2 k1 kc0 c1 c2 c3 c4 c5 c6 c7 c8 c9
Aduki beans	---x---
Beans, fresh green	---------x----
Black soybeans	-------------------x-----------------
Black-eyed peas	---x---
Chickpeas (garbanzo beans)	----x----------
Fava beans (broadbeans)	---x---
Great northern beans	---x---
Green peas, dried	---x---
Kidney beans	---x---
Lentils	-x--------------
Mung beans	---x---
Natto	---x---
Navy beans	----x----------
Peanuts	-------------x-------------
Pinto beans	----x----------
Red beans	---x-----------------
Snow peas, dried	---x---
Soy cheese	-------------x---------------------
Soy milk, natural and fresh	----x------------------------------
Split peas, green or yellow	----x-------
Sprouts, from dried soybeans	---x------
Sprouts, from other dried beans	---------x-------
Tempeh	---x--------------
Tofu, commercial	------------x------------
Tofu, natural nigari	------x------
White beans	----x-------
Yellow beans, with formed beans	---x---
Yellow beans, without formed beans	----------x---

The "x" indicates the over all average of the food and the dashed line indicates the average range of each food. Foods in italics contain a large amount of acid and are acid forming for some people and alkaline forming for others, see pages 37 and 41.

People who have trouble processing foods with a lot of acids may need to reduce or eliminate fruits until their acid-processing ability increases. If fruits are desired, a small amount of unsulfured dried fruit is easier to process than fresh fruits. Soak dried fruits in water for 12 to 24 hours before eating if you have any trouble eating dried fruits. People with a serious disease such as cancer should avoid fruits and foods from other food groups that contain a lot of acids until the disease is cured. These foods are identified in italics in all food charts in this book.

Beans

Beans are a flavorful protein source and a good complement to whole grains. They are another good carbohydrate source and add some fat that is useful for vegetarians and others who are eliminating or reducing their meat intake. Dried beans are mildly acid forming, while beans sprouts are alkaline forming. A chart of beans (and bean products) and their general alkaline-forming and acid-forming effects is on page 40.

Dried beans contain concentrated nutrients that can be difficult for the body to metabolize. Anything that helps in digestive processing moves them in an alkaline-forming direction. Here is a list of factors: "+" indicates an alkaline-forming direction while "–" indicates an acid-forming direction.

1. Quantity: move –1 to –3 if beans are eaten in excess.
2. Quality: move –1 to –3 if beans are pre-cooked, canned, frozen, or preserved in any way.
3. Cooking: move –2 to –4 if refined sugar or other highly acid-forming substances are added to beans during cooking. The values listed for beans are for properly soaked and cooked beans with a small amount of sea salt added.
4. Preparation: move +2 to +4 (or more) if beans are sprouted. Bean sprouts are much easier to digest than cooked beans.

The study and use of dried beans and bean products can be very beneficial. There is one bean, however that requires special attention. Trypsin is an enzyme in the pancreatic juice that helps in processing

Acid and Alkaline of Nuts and Seeds

	Alkaline ← + neutral − → Acid
	k9 k8 k7 k6 k5 k4 k3 k2 k1 kc0 c1 c2 c3 c4 c5 c6 c7 c8 c9
Alfalfa sprouts	-------x----
Almond butter	---x---
Almonds	----------------------x------------
Black walnuts	-----------x-------------------------
Brazil nuts	----------------------------x-----------------------
Cashew butter	-----------------------------------x----------
Cashews	-----------------------------------x----------
Chestnuts	----------------------x-------------
Coconut, dried	------------------------x----
Coconut, fresh	-----------x-----------------
English walnuts	---------------------x------------------
Filberts	--------x------------
Flax seeds	-x---------------
Flour chestnut	---x---
Hazelnuts	-------------------------x-----------------
Macadamia nuts	-----------------------x-
Nut and seed butters	--------x----------
Peanut butter, unsweetened	---x---
Pecans	------------x--------------
Pistachio butter	---------------------------------x-
Pistachios	----------x-------------------------
Pumpkin seeds	----------------------x-----------------
Sesame butter	------------------x-
Sesame seeds, hulled chemically	---x---
Sesame seeds, hulled mechanically	---x---
Sprouts, from most seeds	--------------x----
Sunflower seeds	-x-------------------------
Tahini	----------------------x-

The "x" indicates the over all average of the food and the dashed line indicates the average range of each food. Foods in italics contain a large amount of acid and are acid forming for some people and alkaline forming for others, see pages 37 and 41.

proteins. Soybeans contain a trypsin inhibitor that diminishes the body's ability to process proteins properly. The more soy products one consumes the more this reduction becomes a problem.

There is a way to eliminate the trypsin inhibitor and that is to ferment soybeans with an inoculant. Miso, soy sauce, tofu, tempeh, and natto are examples of soy products with the trypsin inhibitor removed in some way, and they are highly recommended. Soymilk, soy cheese, and soy yogurt are also useful foods but vary greatly in quality.

Advice on soybeans and soy products is available in *The New Whole Foods Encyclopedia* by Rebecca Wood. She does not recommend whole boiled soybeans; highly refined soy products such as soy deli foods from burgers to hot dogs, soy flakes, soy flour, soy grits, soy nuts, soy nut butter; or super refined soy products such as lecithin, soy isolates, soy protein, or textured soy or vegetable protein.

Another very useful book is *Japanese Foods That Heal* by John and Jan Belleme.

Nuts and Seeds

Nuts and seeds are energy foods and a good source of protein and fat for people wanting to avoid or reduce animal foods. Most nuts and seeds are mildly acid forming while sprouts made from nuts and seeds are mildly alkaline forming. Nut butters are harder to digest and are more acid forming than the nuts from which they are made. Seed butters are a bit easier to digest because seeds are less fatty than nuts in general. A chart of organic nuts and seeds and their general alkaline-forming and acid-forming effects is on page 42.

Almonds, technically a fruit, contain cyanidelike substances that have strong medicinal properties, for which they are highly regarded. Peanuts, technically a legume, and peanut butter are very popular worldwide as a protein source although they can be an allergen to many people, especially when chemically altered. Here is a list of factors that move nuts and seeds in an alkaline-forming ("+") or an acid-forming ("–") direction.

Acid and Alkaline of Vegetable Fats and Oils

	Alkaline ← + neutral – → Acid																		
	k9	k8	k7	k6	k5	k4	k3	k2	k1	kc0	c1	c2	c3	c4	c5	c6	c7	c8	c9
Almond oil											-	x	-	-	-	-			
Avocado oil							-	-	x	-	-								
Canola oil (rape seed oil)											-	-	x	-	-	-			
Chestnut oil												-	x	-					
Coconut oil									-	-	x	-	-	-	-	-	-	-	-
Corn oil											-	x	-	-	-	-			
Cottonseed oil																	-	x	-
Flax oil					-	-	x	-	-										
Grape seed oil												-	x	-					
Hazelnut oil															-	x	-		
Hempseed oil, from untreated seeds							-	x	-										
Hydrogenated oil		-	x	-															
Linseed oil					-	x	-												
Macadamia oil									-	-	x	-	-						
Margarine, hydrogenated														-	-	x	-	-	
Margarine, nonhydrogenated							-	x	-										
Olive oil									-	-	x	-	-	-					
Palm kernel oil												-	x	-					
Palm oil													-	-	x	-			
Peanut oil												-	x	-	-	-	-		
Pumpkin seed oil											-	x	-						
Rice bran oil, refined																	-	x	-
Safflower oil, cold pressed									-	-	x	-	-	-	-				
Sesame oil, unrefined											x	-	-	-	-	-			
Soy margarine											x	-	-	-	-	-	-	-	-
Soy oil											-	-	-	-	-	x	-		
Sunflower oil, cold pressed									-	-	x	-	-						
Walnut oil																	-	x	-

The "x" indicates the over all average of the food and the dashed line indicates the average range of each food.

1. Quantity: move −1 to −3 if nuts or seeds are eaten in excess. All fatty nuts aggravate all health problems when eaten in excess.
2. Processing: move −1 to −3 if nuts or seeds are pre-cooked, smoked, or roasted.
3. Quality: move −2 to −4 if nuts or seeds are chemically altered or processed.
4. Production: move −2 to −3 if seeds are hulled chemically and −1 to −2 if hulled mechanically. Whole seeds are always preferred over hulled seeds.
5. Harvesting: move −1 to −2 if nuts or seeds are shelled and are allowed to sit for a long time before eating. Similarly, nut and seed butters become rancid the longer they sit opened before use.
6. Move −1 to −4 if nut or seed butters are sweetened, contain added inferior oil or table salt, or are chemically altered during processing.
7. Move −1 to −2 if the nuts or seeds or their butters are not organic.
8. Move +1 to +2 if nuts or seeds are soaked overnight in distilled water.

The study and use of nuts and seeds can be very beneficial. Flax seeds are the highest source of Omega-3 fatty acids and have many healing properties but should be used in moderation as a raw condiment because they contain prussic acid. Chia seeds, English walnuts, and pumpkin seeds are good sources of Omega-3 fatty acids as well. Sesame seeds are high in calcium but also contain oxalic acid—soaking them overnight removes the oxalic acid and makes the calcium more available to the body. Information on nuts and seeds is available in Rebecca Wood's *The New Whole Foods Encyclopedia.*

Vegetable Fats and Oils

We all need fat and most of us have no problem getting enough fat in our diet unless we intentionally restrict fatty foods. Many foods from nuts and seeds to some grains and beans contain a reasonable amount of fat. Most animal foods contain significant amounts of fat. We use vegetable oils and animal fats (unless animal foods are intentionally avoided) in cooking and as dressings for salads and so on.

Getting enough fat is usually not a problem—it's the quantity

Acid and Alkaline of Animal Foods

	Alkaline ← + neutral – → Acid k9 k8 k7 k6 k5 k4 k3 k2 k1 kc0 c1 c2 c3 c4 c5 c6 c7 c8 c9
Bacon	----X---- (c7)
Butter, clarified (ghee)	-X------------------------ (k3)
Butter, heated (as in cooking)	----X---- (c7)
Butter, processed	-------X------- (c2)
Cheeses, hard	-------X--- (c7)
Cheeses, soft	--------X---- (c3)
Chicken	-----------X----------- (c4)
Egg whites	----X---- (c1)
Egg yolk	----X---- (k2)
Eggs, scrambled or hard-boiled	----X---- (c4)
Fish, cold water	----X---- (c3)
Fish, farmed	----X---- (c7)
Fish, fatty	----X---- (c3)
Fish, lean	----X---- (c3)
Hamburger, beef	----X--- (c7)
Lamb, mutton	-----------X---- (c6)
Lamb, young	----X---- (c3)
Milk, cow's, homogenized, pasteurized	----X------- (c2)
Milk, cow's, raw	--------X-------- (kc0)
Milk shakes, commercial	----X--- (c7)
Pastrami	----X---- (c3)
Pepperoni	----X---- (c3)
Pork	----X---- (c4)
Poultry	-----------X------- (c4)
Sausage	----X--- (c7)
Turkey	-----------X----------- (c4)
Yogurt, aged	----X---- (c3)
Yogurt, plain, fresh	------X----------- (c2)

The "x" indicates the over all average of the food and the dashed line indicates the average range of each food. Foods in italics contain a large amount of acid and are acid forming for some people and alkaline forming for others, see pages 37 and 41.

and type of fat that can be a problem. Still, most fats and unrefined oils are either mildly alkaline forming or mildly acid forming. A chart of unrefined vegetable fats and oils and their general alkaline-forming and acid-forming effects is on page 44.

There are good oils, and there are bad oils, and there are oils that are good used one way and bad if used another way. Research continues. Yesterday's good oil is today's bad oil. Healthy diet advocates are recommending less (or no) deep-fried foods, less saturated fats, and more essential-fatty-acid-rich foods. Essential fatty acids are required in proper proportion for healthy cell functioning. Here is a list of factors that move fats and oils in an acid-forming ("–") direction.

1. Move –3 to –6 if oil is refined. Buy only oils that say unrefined on the label. Refined oils should be avoided at all times.
2. Move –2 to –4 if fats and oils are eaten in excess. Fats and oils aggravate all health problems when eaten in excess.
3. Move –3 to –6 if unrefined oil is heated beyond the temperatue at which it denatures.

The study and proper use of fats and oils can be most beneficial. Flax, hemp, and sunflower oil are rich in essential fatty acids—specifically Omega 3s have a fragile shelf life, and should be kept in the refrigerator in black bottles. Oils made from genetically modified plants should be avoided. Oil may be extracted from many foods and more oils enter the marketplace each year. Look for unrefined oils that have not been subjected to high heat during processing. Complete information on fats and oils is available in *Fat Chance: Surviving the Cholesterol Controversy and Beyond* by Dennis Willmont or *The New Whole Foods Encyclopedia* by Rebecca Wood.

Animal Foods

Most animal foods are rich in protein and fat. Foods like milk, cheese, eggs, and fish are touted by some as promoting health. More poultry and less red meat is a currently popular theory. An increasing number of people from secretaries to world-class athletes are choosing to avoid animal foods completely. This section is for those persons who want to include animal foods in their diets in a healthy way especially with respect to acid and alkaline.

One way to counter an overly acidic internal environment is to increase the amount and strength of alkaline-forming foods. Another way is to decrease the amount and strength of acid-forming foods. Dairy foods are the least acid forming among animal foods. As groups, fish is next, followed by poultry, and finally red meat, which is highly acid forming. A chart of organic, non-chemicalized animal foods (unless noted otherwise) showing effects from slightly alkaline forming to severely acid forming is on page 46.

The complete chart beginning on page 66 includes many more animal products. The quality of animal foods varies greatly and must be considered when choosing which products to buy. Chemicals may be introduced at any time from feeding to processing the end products. Here is a list of factors that move animal foods in an acid-forming ("–") direction.

1. Move –1 to –3 if animals are not organically raised and/or are raised in a factory (are not allowed to run around).
2. Move –2 to –4 if chemicals or sugar are added during processing.
3. Move –2 to –3 if butter or ghee is used for cooking and is subjected to high heat.
4. Move –1 to –2 if cheese has a lot of added table salt.

The study and proper use of animal foods can be very beneficial. Cow's milk is very popular but is the number one food allergen. Goat's milk contains ten times more iron than cow's milk and is easier to digest. Chemical-free cheese from whole, unpasteurized milk is best. Chicken is one of the most chemicalized foods; buy organically fed free-range chickens and other poultry, and purhcase eggs from such animals. Buy fish as fresh as possible. Be aware that some freshwater fish may contain pesticide residues. Most importantly, be certain to neutralize the acid-forming effect of animal foods with plenty of alkaline-forming foods at the same meal.

Sugar and Sweeteners

Most of us like sweets. Most sweets, however, are highly acid forming, especially refined sugar and artificial sweeteners. A diet of primarily meat and sugar usually leads to excess acidity. Vegetarians with excess acidity usually find that the cause is excess refined sugar or artificial sweeteners and/or excess poor quality oils. Another cause is over-eating any foods from vegetables and poor quality oils to grains and beans to meat and sugar.

If sweeteners are used, care needs to be taken to find the best quality and to use them in moderation. The sugar industry is constantly searching for new ways to market their products as "healthful." Many of these products have even found their way into natural health food stores.

Here is a partial list of sweeteners that are best to avoid completely; all are highly to severely acid forming.

Artificial sweeteners	Manitol
Aspartame	Mascouadio sugar
Beet juice, processed	Milled cane
Brown sugar	Molasses, commercial
Cane crystals	Natural milled sugar cane
Corn syrup	Raw cane juice
Dehydrated cane juice	Saccharin
Dextrose	Sorbitol
Dried evaporated cane juice	Sucrose
Fructose	Sugar cane juice (sucanot)
Fruit juice concentrate	Turbinado
Granular fruit sugar	Unrefined cane sugar
Granulated cane juice	White sugar
Invest sugar	Xylitol
Isomol	Yellow D sugar
Malitol	

Acid and Alkaline of Sugar and Sweetners

	Alkaline ← + neutral − → Acid
	k9 k8 k7 k6 k5 k4 k3 k2 k1 kc0 c1 c2 c3 c4 c5 c6 c7 c8 c9
Artificial sweeteners	--------------x-
Barley malt syrup	----------------------x-----------
Beet juice sweetener	----x----
Brown rice syrup, organic	----x------------------
Brown sugar, commercial	-------x----
Candies, sugar	-x----
Carob syrup	----x----
Corn syrup	----x----
Date sugar	-x------------------------------
Fructose	----x-----------
Fruit juice concentrate	----x----
Honey, pasteurized	-x--------------
Honey, raw	-x--------------
Maguey (concentrated cactus juice)	----x----
Maple sugar	----x----
Maple syrup, commercial	-------x-------
Maple syrup, organic	-x-------
Mirin, chemically-processed	----x----
Mirin, traditionally-processed	----x----
Molasses	-------x--------------
Molasses, sulphured	-------x-----------
Pear concentrate	-------x-
Rapadura, commercial	----x----
Rapadura, unrefined (organic)	----x----
Sorghum molasses	----------x-------
Stevia	---------------------------x------------
Sugar cane	----x----
Sugar, white	-------x----

The "x" indicates the over all average of the food and the dashed line indicates the average range of each food.

Barley malt and brown rice syrup come from grains, take longer for the body to process than simple sugars, and may be used in moderation. Sweeteners such as carob, date sugar, honey, maple syrup, rapadura, and sorghum molasses contain a high concentration of sucrose (a simple sugar) but may be used sparingly if desired by people in good health. These products also may be altered.

Here is a list of factors that move sweeteners in the acid-forming ("–") direction.

1. Move –2 to –4 if sucrose or fructose in any form is added or if the sweetener is highly refined or processed.
2. Move –2 to –3 if fruit juice is used as a sweetener and the pulp has been removed—the pulp contains the minerals.
3. Move –2 to –4 if sweeteners are used in excess.

The study and proper use of sweeteners can be most beneficial. These are several healthy alternatives to refined sugar and its many forms. Some people swear by honey and stevia (a sweet herb used as a sweetener). Other people claim they can be harmful and prefer barley malt syrup or brown rice syrup. Still other people prefer rapadura (unrefined, evaporated cane juice used as a sweetener) or organic, unsulphured black strap molasses, or mirin (a fermented sweet rice sweetener). Full information on sweeteners is available in Rebecca Wood's *The New Whole Foods Encyclopedia*.

Beverages

Water is necessary for life and most people drink water daily. Some foods, especially some vegetables and fruit are mostly water. We drink other liquids as well. These beverages originate from a variety of sources from vegetables and herbs to fruits and nuts to grains and beans to dairy foods. The acid-forming or alkaline-forming effect of water and other beverages depends on the source and how it is treated or processed. On the next page, a chart shows beverages and their general alkaline-forming and acid-forming effects.

Because the pH scale is based on the amount of ions in pure water (H_2O), many people believe water is neutral. This simply is not the case. There are many more substances in the water we drink.

Acid and Alkaline of Beverages

	Alkaline ← + neutral – → Acid																		
	k9	k8	k7	k6	k5	k4	k3	k2	k1	kc0	c1	c2	c3	c4	c5	c6	c7	c8	c9
Alcohol, most types																		X	
Almond milk, sweetened												X							
Almond milk, unsweetened								X											
Apple juice, sweetened														X					
Apple juice, unsweetened										X									
Bancha tea								X											
Barley grass juice									X										
Black tea															X				
Carrot juice, with pulp					X														
Carrot juice, without pulp													X						
Coffee, decaffeinated																		X	
Coffee, organic, fresh ground													X						
Coffee, processed, expresso																		X	
Cola drink, sweetened																			X
Fruit juice, naturally sweetened							X												
Fruit juice, sweetened with sugar														X					
Grain coffee (yannoh)								X											
Green tea							X												
Herbal tea									X										
Human milk								X											
Orange juice										X									
Rice milk													X						
Water, carbonated heavily														X					
Water, carbonated slightly													X						
Water, filtered										X									
Water, in plastic bottle													X						
Whiskey																			X
Wine, red or white																	X		

The "x" indicates the over all average of the food and the dashed line indicates the average range of each food. Foods in italics contain a large amount of acid and are acid forming for some people and alkaline forming for others, see pages 37 and 41.

Most tap water is treated and is acid forming. Beverages begin with the alkaline-forming or acid-forming value of their source food. What is done to water during treatment or to beverages in processing moves the alkaline-forming ("+") or acid-forming ("–") effect one direction or the other.

1. Move –2 to –4 if acid-forming elements such as chlorine or fluoride are in or are added to tap water.
2. Move –1 to –3 the more water or other beverages is carbonated.
3. Move +1 to +4 the more alkaline-forming minerals potassium, calcium, magnesium, or iron are in water, unless they are removed during processing.
4. Move –2 to –4 if sugar, sugar substitutes, or chemicals are added to beverages during processing.
5. Move –1 to –3 if consuming poor quality wine or other alcoholic beverages. Getting drunk is severely acid forming.
6. Move –2 to –3 if water or other beverages is purchased in plastic bottles. It is best to avoid cheap plastic bottles

The study and proper use of water can be highly beneficial. Many people filter tap water or bottled water. Bottled water, however, is often just bottled tap water from somewhere else. Filtered water is good if it doesn't contain nitrates, nitrites, or sodium fluoride. Other people find a good, reliable source of well water. It is vitally important to find a good source of water and to drink a proper amount of it each day. A pinch of sea salt in each glass of water is beneficial.

The study of use of other beverages can be equally beneficial. Commercial beverages are dehydrating in effect—drink them sparingly if at all. People who need to reduce acidic wastes would do well to avoid all sugared and carbonated drinks, to increase the proportion of good quality water over other beverages, and to replace acid-forming beverages with homemade vegetable juices that include the pulp. Many alternative beverages to highly processed commercial products may be found in Rebecca Wood's *The New Whole Foods Encyclopedia*.

Summary of Foods

The foods we choose and the way we cook and eat them makes a big difference in how we feel, the amount of energy we have, and the sicknesses we acquire. A healthy internal environment is of primary importance for proper functioning and repair. Here are suggestions based on one's present condition.

For people in perfect health

1. Eat a proportion of 55 to 60 percent alkaline-forming foods to 40 to 45 percent acid-forming foods.
2. Pay attention and remedy any temporary warning signals as they arise.

For people with one or more warning signals (pages 14-16)

1. Eat a proportion of 60 to 65 percent alkaline-forming foods to 35 to 40 percent acid-forming foods until the warning signal is remedied.
2. Avoid masking the problem with medication without tending to the underlying source, especially if the cause is an acid or alkaline imbalance.
3. Choose better quality and more alkaline-forming foods from each food group.

For people with one or more disorders (pages 16-17)

1. Eat a proportion of 65 to 75 percent alkaline-forming foods to 25 to 35 percent acid-forming foods until the disorder is remedied.
2. Realize that most medications are acid forming and are for temporary relief only. If correcting any acid or alkaline imbalance is not enough, make certain the cause is not a nutritional deficiency.
3. Avoid all extremely acid-forming foods from each food group.
4. Choose the least processed foods and beverages and drink a higher proportion of water (with a pinch of sea salt) to other

beverages.
5. Seek medical or other health care provider help when necessary.

For people with serious or life-threatening disease (pages 17-18)

1. Eat a proportion of 70 to 80 percent alkaline-forming foods to 20 to 30 percent acid-forming foods until the disease is remedied.
2. Realize that most medications are acid forming and if taken, must be neutralized with alkaline-forming foods, especially if the underlying cause is excess acidity. Alkaline-forming supplements may be taken for a while but a change in dietary habits is better and more long lasting.
3. Avoid or reduce intake of fruits and other foods high in acid content (in italics in charts) until the disease is remedied.
4. Avoid all chemically processed and sugared foods.
5. Choose the best acid-forming protein and fat sources.
6. Avoid junky oils and all products that contain junky oil.
7. Eat and drink in moderation, except for water. Make certain to drink the right amount of water (with a pinch of sea salt) for your condition.
8. Make unsweetened vegetable drinks at home, and include edible skins.
9. Engage in less acid-forming activities and in more alkaline-forming ones.
10. Seek medical or another health care provider's help when necessary.

The study and use of whole, natural foods can be very beneficial. There is a great variety of healthy foods. Greater reliance on fresh vegetables (including sea vegetables), naturally made pickles and condiments, quality herbs and spices, whole grains, beans, nuts and seeds, and fruits (when one's condition allows) is one way to greater health and an acid and alkaline balanced diet.

The way food is eaten also influences its acid-forming or alkaline-forming effect as does the quantity as shown in the next chapter on lifestyle factors. See also the references on pages 107-109 for further study.

Chapter 4

Lifestyle Factors

Our daily activities, feelings, thoughts, beliefs, and spiritual outlook all have an effect on our internal environment. The effect varies from person to person and needs to be considered when planning one's day. Here is a list of factors and their likely alkaline-forming or acid-forming effects.[1]

Alkaline Forming	Acid Forming
Breathing: practices deep breathing exercises daily and as needed throughout the day	Breathing: often breathes shallowly and doesn't take time to consciously breathe deeply
Sunlight: spends time in the moon light	Sunlight: spends extended periods of time in the sun; ½ hour per day of non-intense sunlight as needed
Eating: eats the proper amount of food (does not overeat) in a relaxed setting and chews food well	Eating: often overeats (eats until stuffed) and/or in a chaotic setting and does not chew food well

[1] These effects were ascertained by the author through research and testing using hydrion paper on saliva and urine samples. These effects have not been documented in scientific studies.

Alkaline Forming	Acid Forming
Drinking: drinks a proper amount of water	Drinking: drinks too little or too much water, thus stressing the kidneys
Organic: eats organic foods and does not eat genetically engineered foods	Organic: regularly eats non-organic vegetables or genetically engineered foods
Eating out: makes one's own meals using the finest (least altered) ingredients and doesn't often eat out in restaurants	Eating out: eats out in restaurants more than once a week or regularly eats packaged processed foods
Drugs: doesn't use marijuana or other mind-altering drugs	Drugs: has used marijuana or other mind-altering drugs in the past year
Movement: physically active	Movement: physically inactive
Exercise: engages in the right amount of exercise such as brisk walks for 20 to 30 minutes each day. Start slowly if beginning exercise after a long period of inactivity, are weak already, or are overly acidic.	Exercise: exercises to exhaustion or engages in stress-producing (that is, life-threatening) activities such as bungee jumping
Bathing: takes cold showers or baths	Bathing: takes hot showers or baths; the longer the more acid-forming

Alkaline Forming	Acid Forming
Environment: lives in a clean environment and away from power lines	Environment: lives in a polluted environment and/or near a cell tower or power lines
Computer: spends little time in front of a computer screen or TV.	Computer: uses a computer or watches TV regularly, especially without regular breaks away from it.
Viruses: rarely, if ever, catches colds or flu viruses because the body's internal environment is not overly acidic to begin with	Viruses: often catches colds and flu viruses because the body is already overly acidic
Jetlag: drinks plenty of water and walks on the plane during long flights; mixing 1 teaspoon of any chlorophyll powder with 8 ounces of water is very beneficial	Jetlag: does nothing to counteract the acid-forming effect of air travel and/or has a fear of flying
Sleep: sleeps well and gets enough deep sleep each night—wakes up quickly and refreshed	Sleep: has trouble falling asleep and tosses and turns all night; has trouble waking up and getting out of bed
Music: listens to music that makes one feel good	Music: listens to music that disrupts or makes one uneasy
Colors: surrounds oneself with colors that foster harmony	Colors: surrounds oneself with colors that impose disharmony

Alkaline Forming	Acid Forming
Accidents: is accident free and has no fear of accidents	Accidents: fears accidents or has an accident with physical trauma (these cause stress both physically and mentally)
Job: loves one's job and feels appreciated	Job: feels overworked and under paid and/or hates one's job
Emotions: deals with emotions appropriately	Emotions: holds negative emotions for long periods of time
Stress: has no stress, worries, or anger and is capable of centering oneself at all times—concentrating on one point (for example the hara area) for 10 to 30 seconds and breathing deeply for 10 to 30 seconds counteracts stress by releasing chyle—an alkaline-forming enzyme	Stress: has stress at home or work; a life-changing event such as a change in marital or financial status, getting fired, or the death of a loved one is very acid forming
Therapies: uses "natural" therapies and the right amount	Therapies: uses medications constantly or too much natural therapy—for example, too much massage can release an excessive amount of stored acids into the system

Alkaline Forming	Acid Forming
Recreational drugs: uses no recreational drugs and avoids cigarettes and second-hand smoke	Recreational drugs: uses mind-altering drugs or smokes cigarettes. Marijuana is severely acid forming.
Ideas: is open to new ideas and people of other cultures	Ideas: is closed minded; tends to say "no" to all new ideas and avoids people form different cultures or backgrounds
Belief: believes in the healing approach (whatever it is) and is confident of a positive result.	Belief: does not have 100 percent confidence in the healing approach and worries about the result.
Compassion: helps others and gives to worthy causes	Compassion: is selfish and overly protective of material possessions
Connection: prays or meditates daily and feels alignment with spirit—that which is beyond scientific understanding, especially when this feeling of alignment leads to a positive outlook on life.	Connection: does not pray or meditate and has a feeling of separation from spirit, especially when this feeling of separation results in a negative outlook on life

We feel the effects in our bodies as our streams get more polluted with pesticides and other chemicals from run off from nearby fields; as our air gets more polluted with aerial spraying, exhaust from traffic, and toxic wastes from factories; and as our cities and lands get more and more overcrowded. As our external environment becomes more acidic, our internal environment also becomes more acidic. Most of us have little control over the external environment, but we have complete control over our internal environment. We can choose less acid-forming foods and lifestyle factors and more alkaline-forming foods and lifestyle factors.

The study and use of calming lifestyle techniques also can be beneficial. Meditation, yoga, deep breathing, and light do-in massage are alkaline forming. Take time to do these or similar practices each day. Any technique that helps relieve stress is helpful in creating a healthy life, as is concentrating more on the alkaline-forming lifestyle factors and less on the acid-forming ones shown in the tables on the preceding pages.

Chapter 5

Acid and Alkaline
Food Tables

My intention when beginning this book was to determine an exact value of acid-forming or alkaline-forming effect for each food. There are so many factors that move a particular food in one direction or the other, however, that this is simply impossible. The following tables are based on research and experience.

First, I consulted every list of acid-forming and alkaline-forming foods that I could find, converting each food value to the value system used in this book. Second, I compared all the values and obtained an average value. For each listing, an "x" is placed in the tables corresponding to that average value.

The range of values found in the various lists is indicated in these tables by dotted lines in the acid-forming or alkaline-forming direction. A small range in the acid-forming or alkaline-forming direction indicates that all values from the various lists provided the same (or a similar) value. The reasoning—if given—was taken into account in all cases in order to evaluate each food listing appropriately.

One cautionary note: many lists found on the Internet had foods that were way out of place according to all other lists with no apparent reason or explanation. In these cases—and in general—I gave more weight to lists from Robert O. Young, PhD; Dr. Theodore A Baroody; Christopher Vasey, ND; Dr. Susan Brown; Annemarie Colbin, PhD; and Herman Aihara. See the resources section on pages 107-109 for more information on these authors and their books.

All foods and products in the following tables are for the highest quality food or product unless otherwise specified. Foods or products that are extremely acid forming should used with discretion or avoided altogether by those seeking a heathy life.

People who have a problem processing foods that contain a large amount of acids should use the more acidic values of all foods, especially those in italics and are advised to avoid foods with brackets around them. All values move in the alkaline-forming ("+") or acid-forming ("–") direction based on many factors as described in Chapters 3 and 4 for each food group. Here is a summary list of some of the main factors. See Chapter 3 for factors specific to each food group.

1. Move +1 to +2 if food is cooked or processed with sea salt.
2. Move –1 to –2 if refined salt is used as it is acid forming and is not recommended.
3. Move –1 to –3 if refined or artificial sugar is added.
4. Move –1 to –2 if food has been pre-cooked, frozen, or canned.
5. Move –2 to –4 if food is grown with chemicals or processed with preservatives.
6. Move –1 to –2 if food is imported and has been fumigated.
7. Move –1 to –4 if food is processed in inferior refined oils.
8. Move –1 to –3 if food is eaten to excess.

Here is a repeat of the table of different food groups for reference. The complete list of foods begins on page 66.

Acid and Alkaline of Food Groups

	Alkaline ← + neutral – → Acid k9 k8 k7 k6 k5 k4 k3 k2 k1 kc0 c1 c2 c3 c4 c5 c6 c7 c8 c9
Grains, whole	`-----------x--------`
Grains, refined	`-----------x--------`
Sprouts from grains and beans	`----------x--------`
Beans, fresh	`-----x------`
Beans, dried	`-------x--------`
Vegetables	`----------x----------`
Sea vegetables	`-------x------`
Pickles, naturally made with sea salt	`----x---------------`
Pickles, commercial	`-----x -----`
Fruits (depends on ability to process)*	`------------x----------------------------`
Nuts and seeds	`----------x----------`
Herbs and spices	`---------x---------`
Vegetable oils	`----------x-----------------------`
Salt, sea	`-------x-------`
Salt, refined table	`-----x-----`
Fish (lean is less acid forming)	`-----------x----------`
Eggs	`--------x--------`
Poultry	`-----------x-------`
Dairy products	`------------x-----------`
Red meats	`-------x------`
Water (depends on composition)	`---------x------------`
Alcohol (natural is less acid forming)	`-------------x-------`
Beverages, sugared	`----x---`
Sugar (refined)	`----x---`
Sweenteners (artifical)	`--x--`
Drugs and medications (most)	`-x-`

The "x" indicates the over all average of the food group and the dashed line indicates the average range of each food group.

* Fruits and other foods that have a large amount of acids can be more difficult to process, especially for people whose health is compromised in any way. Such people will find that these foods are acid forming for them while alkaline forming for others. See pages 37 and 41.

	Alkaline ← + neutral – → Acid k9 k8 k7 k6 k5 k4 k3 k2 k1 kc0 c1 c2 c3 c4 c5 c6 c7 c8 c9
Acetic vinegar	-----x----
Acidophilus milk	----x----
Acorn squash	----x----
Acorns	----x----
Aduki beans	----x----
Agar	----x-------
Alaria	----x----
Alcohol, most types	-----------x----
Ale, dark	----x----
Ale, pale	----x----
Alfalfa sprouts	-------x----
Alfalfa tea	----x----
Algae, blue-green	----x----
Almond butter	----x----
Almond milk, sweetened	-------x----
Almond milk, unsweetened	----x-------
Almond oil	----x---------
Almonds	--------------------x------------
Amaranth	----x------------
Amaranth flour	--------x---------
Amasake pickles	----x----
Amasake, unsweetened	----x----
American cheese, highly processed	-----x----
Anasazi beans	----x----
Angelica	----x----
Anise	----x----
Annatto	----x----
Antibiotics	-----x----
Antihistamines	----x----
Apple butter	-x-------------------------------
Apple cider	----x-----------------------------------

The "x" indicates the over all average of the food group and the dashed line indicates the average range of each food group. Foods in italics contain a large amount of acid and are acid forming for some people and alkaline forming for others, see pages 37 and 41.

	Alkaline ← + neutral – → Acid
	k9 k8 k7 k6 k5 k4 k3 k2 k1 kc0 c1 c2 c3 c4 c5 c6 c7 c8 c9
Apple cider vinegar, raw, unpasteurized	-------x--------------------
Apple juice, sweetened	----------------x----
Apple juice, unsweetened	-x----------------------------
Apples, dried	-x----------------------------
Apples, sour	-x----------------------------
Apples, sweet, unwaxed, organic	-x--
Applesauce, sweetened	------------x-------
Applesauce, unsweetened	-x----------------------------
Apricots, dried, sulfur treated or tart	-x----------------------------
Apricots, dried, sweet	----x-----------------------------------
Apricots, ripe	----x-----------------------------
Apricots, unripe	-x----------------------------
Arame	----x----
Arrowroot powder	----x----
Artichokes, globe	---------------x-------
Artichokes, Jerusalem or Chinese	------x-
Artificial sweeteners	---------------x-
Arugula	----x----
Asafetida	----x----
Asian pears	-------x-------------------------------
Asparagus	--------x--------------
Aspartame	--------------x-
Avocado oil	-------x----
Avocados	----x-------
Bacon	-----x---
Baking chocolate	-----x---
Baking powder	----x----
Baking soda	----x----
Balsamic vinegar	-------x-----------
Bamboo shoots	----x----
Banana smoothie, unsweetened	-x-------

The "x" indicates the over all average of the food group and the dashed line indicates the average range of each food group. Foods in italics contain a large amount of acid and are acid forming for some people and alkaline forming for others, see pages 37 and 41.

	Alkaline ← + neutral – → Acid	
	k9 k8 k7 k6 k5 k4 k3 k2 k1 kc0	c1 c2 c3 c4 c5 c6 c7 c8 c9
Banana squash	----x----	
Bananas	-----------x------------------	
Bananas, dried	-----------x-----------	
Bananas, green		-------x-
Bancha tea	----x----	
Barley flour		----x----
Barley grass juice	------------------x---	
Barley grits (groats)		-------x--------
Barley malt sugar		----------------------x-----------
Barley malt syrup		----------------------x-----------
Barley miso	--------------x-------	
Barley, pearl (hato mugi)		-------x--------
Barley, whole grain		-------x--------
Basil	----x-------	
Basmati rice, brown		----x----
Bass, freshwater		----x-------
Bass, sea		----x----
Bay leaf	----x-------	
Bean sprouts	----------x-----	
Beans, fresh green	----------x----	
Bear		----x-------
Beef		-----x---
Beef bologna		-----x---
Beefsteak leaves, fresh or powdered (from making umeboshi)	----x----	
Beer, dark		--------------x----
Beer, European		----------x-------
Beer, light		----------x-------
Beet greens	----x----	
Beet juice	----x----	
Beet juice sweetener		-----x---

The "x" indicates the over all average of the food group and the dashed line indicates the average range of each food group. Foods in italics contain a large amount of acid and are acid forming for some people and alkaline forming for others, see pages 37 and 41.

	Alkaline ← + neutral − → Acid																		
	k9	k8	k7	k6	k5	k4	k3	k2	k1	kc0	c1	c2	c3	c4	c5	c6	c7	c8	c9
Beets					X														
Bell peppers (sweet, green, or red)					X														
Benzoate (preservative)															X				
Berry juice blend							X												
Birchbark tea												X							
Bison (buffalo)														X					
Bitter melons						X													
Black currents				X															
Black olives, in oil, sundried									X										
Black pepper						X													
Black peppercorns						X													
Black sesame seeds					X														
Black soybeans													X						
Black tea														X					
Black turtle beans											X								
Black walnuts											X								
Black-eyed peas											X								
Blackberries									X										
Blackthorn berries (sloe)								X											
Blue corn											X								
Blue fish														X					
Blue-green algae							X												
Blueberries									X										
Boar, wild														X					
Bok choy							X												
Bolete mushrooms									X										
Bolita beans											X								
Bologna, beef																		X	
Bologna, bratwurst link													X						
Bologna, turkey													X						
Borage							X												

The "x" indicates the over all average of the food group and the dashed line indicates the average range of each food group. Foods in italics contain a large amount of acid and are acid forming for some people and alkaline forming for others, see pages 37 and 41.

	Alkaline ← + neutral – → Acid k9 k8 k7 k6 k5 k4 k3 k2 k1 kc0 c1 c2 c3 c4 c5 c6 c7 c8 c9
Borage oil	----X----
Boullion, mineral (Dr. Bronner's)	----X----
Boysenberries	-X------------------------------
Bran, oat	----X----
Bran pickles, nuka	----X----
Bran, rice	----X----
Bran, wheat	----X----
Bratwurst link bologna	----X----
Brazil nuts	-------------------------X----------------------
Bread, corn, refined	----X----
Bread, corn, unrefined	-------X----
Bread, dark	----X----
Bread, millet, sprouted	----X----
Bread, oat	----X----
Bread, oat, sprouted	----X----
Bread, pumpernickel	----X----
Bread, rice, sprouted	----X----
Bread, rice, whole grain	-------X----
Bread, rye, sprouted	----X----
Bread, white, yeasted	-----X---
Bread, whole wheat	----X----
Bread, whole wheat, sprouted	----X----
Breadfruit	-X-------------------------
Brewer's yeast	----X----
Brick cheese	----X----
Brie cheese, fresh, young, with little fat	----------X-
Brie cheese, ripe, old, with higher fat	-------X----
Brine pickles	----X----
Broccoflower	----X----
Broccoli	--------X----------
Broccoli rabe	----X----

The "x" indicates the over all average of the food group and the dashed line indicates the average range of each food group. Foods in italics contain a large amount of acid and are acid forming for some people and alkaline forming for others, see pages 37 and 41.

	Alkaline ← + neutral – → Acid
	k9 k8 k7 k6 k5 k4 k3 k2 k1 kc0 c1 c2 c3 c4 c5 c6 c7 c8 c9
Broccoli sprouts	----x----
Brown basmati rice	----x----
Brown rice	-------x----
Brown rice cakes (unsalted)	----x----
Brown rice cream	----x----
Brown rice flour	----x-------
Brown rice, puffed cereal	----x----
Brown rice syrup, organic	----x----------------
Brown rice vinegar, traditionally brewed	----x----
Brown sugar, commercial	-------x----
Brussels sprouts	--------------x----
Buckwheat flour	----x----
Buckwheat groats	----------------x----
Buckwheat noodles, (soba, 60 to 80% buckwheat)	----x----
Buffalo	----x-------
Bulgur (cracked wheat)	-------x----
Burdock	----x-------
Burger, veggie, mostly bean	----x----
Burger, veggie, mostly grain	----x-------
Burger, veggie, mostly soy	-----x----
Butter, almond	----x----
Butter beans (lima beans)	--------x------------------
Butter, cashew	--------------------------x------------
Butter, clarified (ghee)	-x---------------------------
Butter, fresh, unsalted	-------x-
Butter, hazelnut	----x----
Butter, heated (as in cooking)	----x----
Butter, nut and seed	-------x----------
Butter, peanut , unsweetened	----x----
Butter, pistachio	--------------------------x-

The "x" indicates the over all average of the food group and the dashed line indicates the average range of each food group. Foods in italics contain a large amount of acid and are acid forming for some people and alkaline forming for others, see pages 37 and 41.

	Alkaline ← + neutral − → Acid
	k9 k8 k7 k6 k5 k4 k3 k2 k1 kc0 c1 c2 c3 c4 c5 c6 c7 c8 c9
Butter, processed	--------x-------
Butter, sesame	--------------x-
Buttermilk, cultured, aged	-------x--------
Buttermilk, fresh	----x----
Butternut squash	----x----
Button mushrooms	----x----
Cabbage	-----------x-------
Cabbage, Chinese	----x----
Cabbage, flowering	----x----
Cabbage, red	----x----
Cabbage, wrapped heart mustard	----x----
Cactus (nopal)	----x----
Calabaga	----x----
Camembert cheese	-----------x-----------
Candies, sugar	-x----
Cannellini beans	----x----
Canola oil (rape seed oil)	----x-------
Canola seeds	----x----
Cantaloupe, melons	----x-----------------------------------
Capers	----x----
Caraway seeds	----x----
Carbonated soft drinks	-x----
Carbonated water, heavy	-------x----
Carbonated water, slight	----x-------
Cardamon seeds	----x----
Carob powder	------x-----------------------------------
Carob syrup	----x----
Carp	----x-------
Carrot juice, with pulp	----x----
Carrot juice, without pulp	----x----
Carrots, commercial (canned)	------------------x--------

The "x" indicates the over all average of the food group and the dashed line indicates the average range of each food group. Foods in italics contain a large amount of acid and are acid forming for some people and alkaline forming for others, see pages 37 and 41.

	Alkaline ← + neutral – → Acid
	k9 k8 k7 k6 k5 k4 k3 k2 k1 kc0 c1 c2 c3 c4 c5 c6 c7 c8 c9
Carrots, organic	--------x-------
Casein, milk protein	----x----
Cashew butter	-------------------------x-----------
Cashews	-------------------------x-----------
Castor oil	-----x----
Catfish	----x----
Catsup (ketchup), sugared	----x-------
Cauliflower	----x-------
Cayenne pepper (capsicum)	-------x--------------
Celeriac	----x----
Celery	---------x--------
Celery juice	----x----
Celery seeds	----x----
Cereals, flaked whole grain	----x----
Chamomile	----x----
Chamomile tea	----x----
Chard (Swiss chard)	-----------x-----------------------
Chayote	----x----
Cheddar cheese, aged	----x----
Cheese, American, highly processed	-----x----
Cheese, soy	-----------------x-----------------------
Cheeses, hard	---------x-----------
Cheeses, hard, stronger flavor	----x----
Cheeses, homogenized	-----x---
Cheeses, medium, from unpasteurized milk	---------------x-
Cheeses, mild, from unpasteurized milk	-------------x-
Cheeses, sharp, from unpasteurized milk	-------------------x-
Cheeses, soft	-------x----
Cheeses, soft, fresh, well-drained	-x--------------
Cheeses, soft, unripened	---------------x-

The "x" indicates the over all average of the food group and the dashed line indicates the average range of each food group. Foods in italics contain a large amount of acid and are acid forming for some people and alkaline forming for others, see pages 37 and 41.

Acid Alkaline Companion

Food	Alkaline ← + neutral – → Acid
	k9 k8 k7 k6 k5 k4 k3 k2 k1 kc0 c1 c2 c3 c4 c5 c6 c7 c8 c9
Chemical additives	----x
Cherimoya	----------------------x-
Cherries, ground	----x-----------------------
Cherries, sour	-x---------------------------
Cherries, sweet	-------x-----------------------
Chervil	----x----
Chestnut flour	----x----
Chestnut oil	----x----
Chestnuts, dry-roasted	----------------------x------------
Chestnuts, water	----x----
Chia seeds	----x----
Chia sprouts	----x----
Chicken	-----------x-----------
Chickpeas (garbanzo beans)	---x-----------
Chicory	-----------x-----------
Chili pepper	----x----
Chili peppers, red	----x----
Chinese broccoli	----x----
Chinese cabbage	----x----
Chinese winter melon	----x----
Chives	----x-----------
Chocolate	-----x----
Chocolate, hot	-------x----
Chocolate milk, whole	-------x----
Chuba iriko (small dried fish)	----x----
Cider, apple	----x-----------------------------
Cigarettes, roll your own	-----x----
Cigarettes, tailor made	----x-------
Cilantro	----x-------
Cinnamon	----x-----------
Citron	-----------x-----------------------

The "x" indicates the over all average of the food group and the dashed line indicates the average range of each food group. Foods in italics contain a large amount of acid and are acid forming for some people and alkaline forming for others, see pages 37 and 41.

	Alkaline ← + neutral – → Acid
	k9 k8 k7 k6 k5 k4 k3 k2 k1 kc0 c1 c2 c3 c4 c5 c6 c7 c8 c9
Citrus fruit, most	--------X--------------------------------------
Citrus peel (zest)	----X----
Clams	----X----
Clarified butter, ghee	-X-------------------------
Clementines (citrus)	-X--------------------------
Clover tea	----X----
Cloves	----X----
Cocoa drink	-----X---
Cocoa powder	-----X---
Cocoa powder, European (alkali-processed)	----X----
Coconut, dried	------------------------X----
Coconut, fresh	-----------X-----------
Coconut milk, sweetened	----X----
Coconut milk, unsweetened	----X----
Coconut oil	--------X------------------------
Cod	----X----
Cod liver oil	----X--------
Coffee, decaffeinated	-----------X----
Coffee, instant	----X
Coffee, Kono	----X----
Coffee, organic, fresh ground	-----------X--------------
Coffee, processed, expresso	-----------X----
Coffee substitute, roasted grains (with chicory)	----X---------
Cola drink, sweetened	-X---
Colby cheese	----X----
Cold cuts	-----X---
Collard greens	---------X--------
Comfrey tea, leaves	----X----
Comfrey tea, roots	----X----

The "x" indicates the over all average of the food group and the dashed line indicates the average range of each food group. Foods in italics contain a large amount of acid and are acid forming for some people and alkaline forming for others, see pages 37 and 41.

	Alkaline ← + neutral – → Acid																	
	k9	k8	k7	k6	k5	k4	k3	k2	k1	kc0	c1	c2	c3	c4	c5	c6	c7	c8	c9
Coriander leaf (cilantro)					X														
Coriander seeds								X											
Corn, blue												X							
Corn bread, refined																		X	
Corn bread, unrefined													X						
Corn chips, baked																	X		
Corn chips, deep fried																			X
Corn flakes, unsweetened																	X		
Corn grits																	X		
Corn nuts																		X	
Corn oil													X						
Corn, puffed																X			
Corn, sweet (corn on the cob)						X													
Corn syrup																			X
Corn tortillas																	X		
Corn, whole (yellow or white, maize)														X					
Corned beef																			X
Cornmeal														X					
Cottage cheese														X					
Cottonseed meal																			X
Cottonseed oil																			X
Couscous, white flour																		X	
Couscous, whole wheat flour																	X		
Crab																	X		
Cracked wheat, bulgur																X			
Crackers, rye (unrefined, unsalted)															X				
Crackers, unrefined rye												X							
Crackers, white flour																		X	
Crackers, whole grain																X			
Crackers, whole wheat																X			
Cranberries															X				

The "x" indicates the over all average of the food group and the dashed line indicates the average range of each food group. Foods in italics contain a large amount of acid and are acid forming for some people and alkaline forming for others, see pages 37 and 41.

Food	Alkaline ← + neutral – → Acid
	k9 k8 k7 k6 k5 k4 k3 k2 k1 kc0 c1 c2 c3 c4 c5 c6 c7 c8 c9
Cranberry beans	----x---- (c3)
Crayfish	----x---- (c6)
Cream cheese	----x---- (c4)
Cream, fresh, processed	----x---- (c3)
Cream, fresh, raw	-----x---- (c0)
Cream of rice	----x---- (c4)
Cream of wheat, unrefined	----x---- (c4)
Cream, sour	----x---- (c3)
Creme fraiche	----x---- (c3)
Cress, fresh garden	----x---- (k3)
Crookneck squash	----x---- (k4)
Crustaceans	----x---- (c7)
Cucumbers	-----------x------- (k3)
Cumin seeds	----x------- (k3)
Curd cheese	----x---- (c4)
Currents, black, white, or yellow	-x-------------------------- (k4)
Currents, red	-----------x-------------------- (k2)
Currents, Zante	-x-------------------------- (k4)
Curry powder	-x------------- (k1)
Dahia, roasted (DaCopa)	----x---- (k3)
Daikon greens	----x---- (k3)
Daikon pickles (takuwan)	----x---- (k6)
Daikon radish	----x------- (k5)
Dal	----x---- (c6)
Dandelion greens	-----------x---- (k3)
Dandelion roots	----x---- (k3)
Dandelion tea	----x---- (k3)
Date sugar	-x-------------------------- (k1)
Dates, dried	----x-------------------------- (k4)
Dates, fresh	-------x------------------- (k3)
Delicata squash	----x---- (k4)

The "x" indicates the over all average of the food group and the dashed line indicates the average range of each food group. Foods in italics contain a large amount of acid and are acid forming for some people and alkaline forming for others, see pages 37 and 41.

	Alkaline ← + neutral − → Acid
	k9 k8 k7 k6 k5 k4 k3 k2 k1 kc0 c1 c2 c3 c4 c5 c6 c7 c8 c9
Dewberries (like blackberries)	----x-------------------------
Dextrose	-----x----
Dill leaves	----x----
Dill pickles, homemade with sea salt	----x----
Dill pickles, with apple cider vinegar	----x----
Dill seeds	----x----
Drugs, most	-x----
Duck eggs	--------x--------
Duck, wild	-----------x-----------
Dulse	----x----
Egg noodles, white flour	-----x----
Egg whites	----x----
Egg yolk	----x----
Eggplant	----x----------------------
Eggs, duck	--------x--------
Eggs, quail	-------x------------
Eggs, scrambled or hard-boiled	----x----
Eggs, whole, chicken	-x--------------
Elephant garlic	----x----
Elk	----x----
Endive	--------x--------------
English walnuts	--------------x------------------
Epazote, dried	----x----
Epazote, fresh	----x----
Equal, sweetener	-----x----
Escarole	----x----
Evening primrose oil	----x----
Farina	----x----
Fava beans (broadbeans)	----x----
Fennel leaves	----x----
Fennel seeds	--------x-------

The "x" indicates the over all average of the food group and the dashed line indicates the average range of each food group. Foods in italics contain a large amount of acid and are acid forming for some people and alkaline forming for others, see pages 37 and 41.

	Alkaline ← + neutral – → Acid k9 k8 k7 k6 k5 k4 k3 k2 k1 kc0 c1 c2 c3 c4 c5 c6 c7 c8 c9
Fenugreek	----x----
Figs, dried	----------x-------------------------
Figs, fresh	-x--------------------------
Filberts	-------x---------------
Fish, cold water	----x----
Fish, farmed	----x----
Fish, fatty	----x----
Fish, lean	----x----
Fish oil	---------------------x-
Fish, wild	----x----
Flageolet	----x----
Flax oil	-------x----
Flax seeds	-x--------------
Flounder	-------x--------
Flour, amaranth	--------x--------
Flour, barley	----x----
Flour, brown rice	----x-------
Flour, buckwheat	----x----
Flour, chestnut	----x----
Flour, millet	---x------------------
Flour, oat	------------------------x----
Flour, rye	----x----
Flour, triticale	----x-------
Flour, white wheat	----x----
Flour, whole wheat	----x----
Flowering cabbage	----x----
Fowl, game birds	-------x----
Frankfurters (hot dogs), beef	-----x----
Frankfurters (hot dogs), pork	----x----
Frankfurters (hot dogs), turkey	----x-------
Frankfurters, soy and bean	----x----

The "x" indicates the over all average of the food group and the dashed line indicates the average range of each food group. Foods in italics contain a large amount of acid and are acid forming for some people and alkaline forming for others, see pages 37 and 41.

	Alkaline ← + neutral – → Acid																	
	k9	k8	k7	k6	k5	k4	k3	k2	k1	kc0	c1	c2	c3	c4	c5	c6	c7	c8	c9
Fried foods, processed																		x	
Fructose											x								
Fruit conserves, homemade, without sugar							x												
Fruit conserves, with sugar or corn syrup																x			
Fruit juice concentrate															x				
Fruit juice, naturally sweetened							x												
Fruit juice, sweetened with sugar														x					
Fruit, pickled											x								
Fruit smoothie, sweetened											x								
Fruits, tropical			x																
Galangal					x														
Garbanzo beans (chickpeas)											x								
Garlic				x															
Gelatin, in water and sugared															x				
Gelatin, in water only												x							
Gelatin with fruit					x														
Gelatin with vegetables								x											
Ghee (clarified butter)							x												
Gin																		x	
Ginger, powdered					x														
Ginger root, fresh			x																
Ginger tea					x														
Ginseng root					x														
Ginseng tea, leaves						x													
Ginseng tea, roots							x												
Goat																x			
Goat cheese										x									
Goat's milk, homogenized										x									
Goat's milk, raw						x													

The "x" indicates the over all average of the food group and the dashed line indicates the average range of each food group. Foods in italics contain a large amount of acid and are acid forming for some people and alkaline forming for others, see pages 37 and 41.

Food	Alkaline ← + neutral – → Acid k9 k8 k7 k6 k5 k4 k3 k2 k1 kc0 c1 c2 c3 c4 c5 c6 c7 c8 c9
Gold nugget squash	----x----
Gomashio (sesame salt)	----x----
Goose	----x----
Gooseberries	-x---------------------------
Gouda cheese	----x-
Gourds, edible	----x----
Grain coffee (yannoh)	----x------------
Granular sugar, fruit	----x----
Granulated sugar, white	-----x----
Grape juice	-x-------------
Grape seed oil	----x----
Grapefruit	-x------------------------------
Grapefruit juice	-x------------------------------
Grapes, less sweet	-x---------------------------
Grapes, seedless	----x------------------------
Grapes, sour	----x----------------------
Grapes, sweet	-x---------------------------
Great northern beans	----x----
Green beans	----------x----
Green bell peppers	----x----
Green onion (scallions)	----x-------
Green peas, dried	----x----
Green peas, fresh	----x----
Green soybeans (edamame)	----x----
Green tea	-----------x-------------
Grits, corn	----x----
Grits (groats), barley	-------x--------
Grits, soy	----x----
Groats, buckwheat	----------------x----
Ground cherries	----x-------------------
Grouper	----x----

The "x" indicates the over all average of the food group and the dashed line indicates the average range of each food group. Foods in italics contain a large amount of acid and are acid forming for some people and alkaline forming for others, see pages 37 and 41.

	Alkaline ← + neutral – → Acid k9 k8 k7 k6 k5 k4 k3 k2 k1 kc0 c1 c2 c3 c4 c5 c6 c7 c8 c9
Guavas	-X------------------:--------
Haddock	----X----
Halibut	----X----
Ham, pork	----X----
Ham, turkey	----X----
Hamburger, beef	-----X---
Hamburger, turkey	----X----
Hazelnut butter	----X----
Hazelnut oil	----X----
Hazelnuts	--------------------X------------------
Hempseed oil, imported and from untreated seeds	----X----
Herbal tea	------------------X----
Herbs, leafy green	-------X----
Herring	----X-------
Herring, pickled	----X----
Hiziki	----X----
Hokkaido pumpkin	----X----
Honey, pasteurized	-X--------------
Honey, raw	-X------------
Honeydew melons	----X--
Hops	-----X---
Horseradish	----X---------------------
Horsetail tea	-X-------
Hot chocolate	-------X----
Hot dogs, beef	-----X---
Hot dogs, pork	----X----
Hot dogs, soy	-----X---
Hot dogs, turkey	----X-------
Hubbard squash	----X----
Human breast milk	--------------X-

The "x" indicates the over all average of the food group and the dashed line indicates the average range of each food group. Foods in italics contain a large amount of acid and are acid forming for some people and alkaline forming for others, see pages 37 and 41.

	Alkaline ← + neutral – → Acid
	k9 k8 k7 k6 k5 k4 k3 k2 k1 kc0 c1 c2 c3 c4 c5 c6 c7 c8 c9
Hydrogenated oil	----x---- (k5)
Ice cream	-------x---- (c6)
Invert sugar	-----x--- (c7)
Irish moss seaweed	-------x---- (k4)
Isomol	-----x--- (c7)
Jacob's cattle bean	-x------- (c1)
Jam, sugared	-----x--- (c7)
Japonica rice	----x---- (k2)
Jellies, sugared	-----x--- (c7)
Jerusalem artichokes	-------x- (k3)
Jicama	-------x---- (k3)
Jinenjo	----x---- (k5)
Juniper berry	----x---- (k2)
Kabocha squash	----x---- (k5)
Kale	---------x-------- (k5)
Kamut cereal	----x---- (c4)
Kanten (agar)	----x------- (k7)
Karengo	----x---- (k7)
Kasha (buckwheat groats)	----------------x---- (c1)
Kefir	----x----------- (c2)
Kelp (kombu, sea palm, wakame, etc.)	----x---- (k9)
Ketchup, natural, homemade	----x---- (k3)
Ketchup, refined, sugared	----x------- (c4)
Kidney beans	----x---- (c1)
Kielbasa sausage	----x---- (c4)
Kiwano	-------x------------------------- (k5)
Kiwis (kiwifruit)	-----------x--------------------------------- (k5)
Knockwurst sausage link	----x---- (c4)
Kohlrabi	---------------x------- (k5)
Kombu	----x---- (k9)
Kombucha	-----------------------------------x- (c1)

The "x" indicates the over all average of the food group and the dashed line indicates the average range of each food group. Foods in italics contain a large amount of acid and are acid forming for some people and alkaline forming for others, see pages 37 and 41.

	Alkaline ← + neutral – → Acid
	k9 k8 k7 k6 k5 k4 k3 k2 k1 kc0 c1 c2 c3 c4 c5 c6 c7 c8 c9
Kono coffee	----x----
Kudzu root	----x----
Kudzu tea	----x----
Kumquats	----x-------------------------
Lactobacillus acidophilus	----x----
Lactobacillus bifidus	----x----
Lamb, mutton	-----------x----
Lamb, young	----x----
Lamb's-quarters	----x----
Lard	-------x--------
Lavender	----x----
Leeks	----x----
Legumes, general	--------x-------
Lemon balm	----x----
Lemon grass	----x----
Lemon juice	-x--
Lemon peel (zest)	----x----
Lemon water	-x-------------------------
Lemons	----x-------------------------------
Lentils	-------------x----
Lettuce, iceberg	----x----
Lettuce, loose leaf	--------x----
Lettuce, romaine	--------x----
Licorice root	----x----
Lima beans	--------x---------------
Lime juice	-x-----------------------------
Lime peel (zest)	----x----
Limes	-x-----------------------
Linden tea	----x----
Linguine, white flour	----x----
Linseed oil	----x----

The "x" indicates the over all average of the food group and the dashed line indicates the average range of each food group. Foods in italics contain a large amount of acid and are acid forming for some people and alkaline forming for others, see pages 37 and 41.

	Alkaline ← + neutral – → Acid
	k9 k8 k7 k6 k5 k4 k3 k2 k1 kc0 c1 c2 c3 c4 c5 c6 c7 c8 c9
Liquor, hard	----x
Liquor, malt, dark	----x----
Liquor, malt, pale	----x----
Liver, beef or chicken	-------x----
Liverwurst	-------x----
Lobster	-----x---
Loganberries	-x--------------------------
Loofah	----x----
Lotus root	-------x----
Lotus root tea	----x----
Lotus seeds	----x----
Lovage	----x----
Luncheon meats	-----------x----
Lupine (bean pasta)	----x----
Macadamia nuts	--------------x-
Macadamia oil	--------x--------
Macaroni and cheese	----x---
Macaroni, white flour	----x----
Macaroni, whole wheat flour	----x----
Mace	----x----
Mache	----x----
Mackerel	----x-------
Maguey (concentrated cactus juice)	----x----
Maize	-------x--------
Malitol	-----x---
Malt	-----x---
Malt liquor, dark	----x----
Malt liquor, pale	----x----
Mandarins	-----------x--------------------------
Mangoes	-----------x--------------------------
Mangoes, dried	-x--------------------------

The "x" indicates the over all average of the food group and the dashed line indicates the average range of each food group. Foods in italics contain a large amount of acid and are acid forming for some people and alkaline forming for others, see pages 37 and 41.

Acid Alkaline Companion

	Alkaline ← + neutral − → Acid																		
	k9	k8	k7	k6	k5	k4	k3	k2	k1	kc0	c1	c2	c3	c4	c5	c6	c7	c8	c9
Mannitol																	x		
Maple sugar														x					
Maple syrup, commercial															x				
Maple syrup, organic												x							
Marijuana																			x
Margarine, hydrogenated															x				
Margarine, vegetable (nonhydrogenated)									x										
Marjoram				x															
Mate						x													
Mayonnaise, natural, homemade									x										
Mayonnaise, refined, sugared														x					
Meat, red																		x	
Meat, white															x				
Medications, most																			x
Mello miso						x													
Melons, cantaloupe		x																	
Melons, honeydew		x																	
Melons, watermelon		x																	
Milk, acidophilus									x										
Milk, almond, sweetened														x					
Milk, almond, unsweetened									x										
Milk, coconut, sweetened															x				
Milk, coconut, unsweetened											x								
Milk, cow's, homogenized, pasteurized													x						
Milk, cow's, raw										x									
Milk, cow's, ultra-pasteurized															x				
Milk, goat's, homogenized, pasteurized													x						
Milk, goat's, raw									x										
Milk, human breast											x								
Milk, oat, homemade														x					
Milk protein, casein														x					

The "x" indicates the over all average of the food group and the dashed line indicates the average range of each food group. Foods in italics contain a large amount of acid and are acid forming for some people and alkaline forming for others, see pages 37 and 41.

	Alkaline ← + neutral − → Acid
	k9 k8 k7 k6 k5 k4 k3 k2 k1 kc0 c1 c2 c3 c4 c5 c6 c7 c8 c9
Milk, rice	-------X----
Milk shakes, commercial	-----X----
Milk, skim (nonfat)	----X----
Milk, soy	--X-
Milk, whole, chocolate-flavored	----X----
Millet	----X----------------------------
Millet bread, sprouted	----X----
Millet flour	---X------------------
Millet, puffed	---X------------------
Mineral water, carbonated heavy	-------X----
Mineral water, carbonated slight	----X-------
Mineral water, non-carbonated	----------------------------X-
Mint	----X----
Mint tea	----X-----------
Mirin, chemically-processed	-----X---
Mirin, traditionally-processed	----X----
Miso, barley	---------------X-------
Miso, mello	-------X----
Miso, most kinds	---------------X-------
Miso pickles	----X----
Miso, rice	---------------X-------
Miso, soybean	---------------X-------
Mizuna	----X----
Molasses	-------X---------------
Molasses, sulphured	-------X-----------
Mollusks	----X----
Monosodium glutamate (MSG)	-X-------
Monterey jack cheese	----X----
Morels (mushrooms)	-------X----
Mozzarella cheese	----X----
Mu tea	-------X----

The "x" indicates the over all average of the food group and the dashed line indicates the average range of each food group. Foods in italics contain a large amount of acid and are acid forming for some people and alkaline forming for others, see pages 37 and 41.

Food	Alkaline ← + neutral − → Acid k9 k8 k7 k6 k5 k4 k3 k2 k1 kc0 c1 c2 c3 c4 c5 c6 c7 c8 c9
Muenster cheese	-------X----
Mulberries	-X----------------------
Mung beans	----X----
Mushrooms, bolete	----X---------------------
Mushrooms, morels or truffles	-------X----
Mushrooms, reishi	----X----
Mushrooms, shiitake	--------X----
Mushrooms, white (button)	----X--------------
Muskmelon (cantaloupe)	----X----------------------------
Mussels	----X-------
Mustard greens	---------X--------
Mustard, natural, stone-ground (yellow or green)	------------------X-----
Mustard, refined, artificially-flavored or prepared	-------X----
Mustard seeds	----X----
Mutton	-----------X----
Natto	----X----
Navy beans	---X-----------
Nectarines	-------X----------------------
Nigella	----X----
Noodles, buckwheat (soba, 100% buckwheat)	----X----
Noodles, buckwheat (soba, 60 to 80% buckwheat)	----X----
Noodles, egg, white flour	-----X----
Noodles, from white flour	----X----
Noodles, from whole grains	-------X--------
Noodles, whole wheat (udon or somen)	----X----
Nori (seaweed)	----X----
Nuña (bean popcorn)	----X----

The "x" indicates the over all average of the food group and the dashed line indicates the average range of each food group. Foods in italics contain a large amount of acid and are acid forming for some people and alkaline forming for others, see pages 37 and 41.

	Alkaline ← + neutral – → Acid																	
	k9	k8	k7	k6	k5	k4	k3	k2	k1	kc0	c1	c2	c3	c4	c5	c6	c7	c8	c9
Nut and seed butters														x					
Nutmeg												x							
Nutra Sweet																		x	
Nutritional yeast								x											
Oat bran														x					
Oat bread														x					
Oat bread, sprouted													x						
Oat flour													x						
Oat milk, homemade														x					
Oats, rolled (oatmeal), sweetened															x				
Oats, rolled (oatmeal), unsweetened													x						
Oats, steel-cut											x								
Oats, whole											x								
Ohsawa coffee										x									
Okara											x								
Okra					x														
Olive oil										x									
Olives, black (sundried and packed in oil)									x										
Olives, green									x										
Olives, pickled											x								
Olives, ripe								x											
Olives, ripe, in brine or vinegar										x									
Onions					x														
Onions, green (scallions)			x																
Oolong tea											x								
Orach				x															
Orange juice								x											
Orange peel (zest)		x																	
Orange roughy														x					
Oranges						x													
Oranges, mandarin				x															

The "x" indicates the over all average of the food group and the dashed line indicates the average range of each food group. Foods in italics contain a large amount of acid and are acid forming for some people and alkaline forming for others, see pages 37 and 41.

	Alkaline ← + neutral – → Acid k9 k8 k7 k6 k5 k4 k3 k2 k1 kc0 c1 c2 c3 c4 c5 c6 c7 c8 c9
Oregano	----X-------
Oysters	--------X----
Palm kernel oil	----X----
Palm oil	-------X----
Pancakes, white flour	----X---
Papaya	--------X--------------------------------
Paprika	-----------X-----------
Parmesan cheese	----X----
Parsley	-----------X-----------
Parsley juice	-----------X-----------
Parsley root	----X----
Parsnips	--------------X-------
Passion fruit	----X----------------------
Pasta, bean (lupine)	----X----
Pasta, buckwheat (soba, 100% buck- wheat)	----X----
Pasta, buckwheat (soba, 60 to 80% buckwheat)	----X----
Pasta, from white flour	----X----
Pasta, from whole grains	-------X--------
Pasta sauce, tomato without meat	----X----
Pasta, whole wheat (udon or somen)	----X----
Pastrami	----X----
Patty pan squash	----X----
Peas, pigeon	----X----
Peaches	----X----------------------
Peaches, dried	----X----------------------
Peanut butter, unsweetened	----X----
Peanut oil	---X-------------------
Peanuts	--------------X---------------
Pear concentrate	-------X-

The "x" indicates the over all average of the food group and the dashed line indicates the average range of each food group. Foods in italics contain a large amount of acid and are acid forming for some people and alkaline forming for others, see pages 37 and 41.

	Alkaline ← + neutral – → Acid
	k9 k8 k7 k6 k5 k4 k3 k2 k1 kc0 c1 c2 c3 c4 c5 c6 c7 c8 c9
Pear juice	----x----
Pearl barley (hato mugi)	-------x--------
Pears, Asian	-------x-----------------------------------
Pears, dried	-x--------------------------
Pears, less sweet	----x-------------------------------
Pears, sweet	----x------------------------------
Peas, black-eyed	----x----
Peas, fresh green	-----------x---------------
Peas, snow	----x-------------------------------
Peas, split, green, or yellow	---x--------
Pecans	------------x--------------
Pepino	-x--------------------------
Pepper, black	----x----
Pepper, cayenne	--------x--------------
Pepper, chili	----x----
Pepperoni	----x----
Peppers, red hot chili	--------x-------
Peppers, sweet, green, red, or bell	-------x-------
Perch, freshwater	----x-------
Perch, sea (white)	----x----
Perilla	----x----
Persimmon juice	-------------------------x-
Persimmons	-----------x-------------------------
Pheasant	----x----
Phosphoric acid, flavoring	-----x----
Pickles, amasake	----x----
Pickles, bran	----x----
Pickles, brine	----x----
Pickles, daikon (takuwan)	----x----
Pickles, dill, homemade	----x----
Pickles, dill, with apple cider vinegar	----x----

The "x" indicates the over all average of the food group and the dashed line indicates the average range of each food group. Foods in italics contain a large amount of acid and are acid forming for some people and alkaline forming for others, see pages 37 and 41.

	Alkaline ← + neutral − → Acid
	k9 k8 k7 k6 k5 k4 k3 k2 k1 kc0 c1 c2 c3 c4 c5 c6 c7 c8 c9
Pickles, miso	`----x----`
Pickles, sake	`-x-------`
Pickles, sea salt	`----x----`
Pickles, sour, commercial	`----x----`
Pickles, soy sauce	`----x----`
Pickles, sweet, with white sugar and vinegar	`----x-------`
Pickles, umeboshi	`----x----`
Pigeon peas	`----x----`
Pike	`----x----`
Pilpil	`----x----`
Pimento	`----x----`
Pine nuts (pignolis)	`-------------------------x-`
Pineapple juice	`-------x----------------------`
Pineapples	`--------------x----------------------`
Pineapples, dried	`-x------------------------`
Pink beans	`----x----`
Pinto beans	`---x-----------`
Pistachio butter	`-------------------------x------------`
Pistachios	`-----------x----------------------`
Plantain	`-----------x-----------`
Plums	`----------x------------------`
Plums, greengage	`---------x--------------------`
Plums, umeboshi	`----x--------`
Pollock	`----x----`
Pomegranates	`-----------x------------------------`
Popcorn	`----x----`
Poppy seeds	`----x----`
Pork	`----x----`
Pork sausage	`----x----`
Potassium salt	`----x----`

The "x" indicates the over all average of the food group and the dashed line indicates the average range of each food group. Foods in italics contain a large amount of acid and are acid forming for some people and alkaline forming for others, see pages 37 and 41.

	Alkaline ← + neutral – → Acid
	k9 k8 k7 k6 k5 k4 k3 k2 k1 kc0 c1 c2 c3 c4 c5 c6 c7 c8 c9
Potato chips, baked	----x---- (k4)
Potato chips, fried	-----x--- (c8)
Potatoes, French fried, commercial	-----x--- (c8)
Potatoes, French fried, homemade (with skins)	--------------x---- (k5)
Potatoes, French fried, homemade (without skins)	----x---- (c3)
Potatoes, sweet	-------x---- (k6)
Potatoes, taro	-----------x----------- (k5)
Potatoes, with skins	-------x----------- (k6)
Potatoes, without skins	-x----------------- (c1)
Poultry	-----------x------- (c5)
Preservatives (benzoate)	--------x---- (c4)
Prickly pears	-x------------------------- (k5)
Primrose oil	-------x---- (k5)
Processed cheese	-----x--- (c8)
Provolone cheese	----x---- (c4)
Prunes	----------------------x---------------- (kc0/c1)
Psychedelic drugs	x (c9)
Psychotropics	----x---- (c6)
Psyllium	----x---- (k3)
Puddings, sugared	-----x--- (c8)
Pumpernickel bread	----x---- (c5)
Pumpkin	----x-------- (k3)
Pumpkin seed oil	----x---- (c3)
Pumpkin seeds	--------------------x------------------ (kc0)
Quail eggs	-------x------------ (k2)
Quince	-x--------------------------------- (k5)
Quinoa	----x------------ (c1)
Rabbit	---------------x-------- (c6)
Radish, daikon	----x------- (k4)

The "x" indicates the over all average of the food group and the dashed line indicates the average range of each food group. Foods in italics contain a large amount of acid and are acid forming for some people and alkaline forming for others, see pages 37 and 41.

	Alkaline ← + neutral − → Acid
	k9 k8 k7 k6 k5 k4 k3 k2 k1 kc0 c1 c2 c3 c4 c5 c6 c7 c8 c9
Radish seed sprouts	-------x-------
Radishes	-----------x-----------
Raisins	-------x------------------
Ramp	----x----
Rapadura, commercial	-----x---
Rapadura, unrefined (organic)	----x----
Raspberries	----------------------x------------------------
Raspberry tea	----x----------------------------
Rattlesnake beans	----x----
Red beans	---x------------------
Red bell peppers	-------x-------
Red cabbage	----x----
Red chili peppers	----x----
Red meat	-----x---
Red snapper	----x-------
Red tea	---x--------
Red wine	----x-------
Red wine vinegar	-------x----
Reishi mushrooms	----x----
Rhubarb	----------------x-----------
Rice bran	----x----
Rice bran oil, refined	----x----
Rice bread, refined	------x-
Rice bread, sprouted	----x----
Rice bread, whole grain	-------x----
Rice, brown	-------x----
Rice, brown basmati	----x----
Rice, brown, puffed cereal	----x----
Rice cakes, brown (unsalted)	----x----
Rice crackers, unrefined	----x----
Rice cream, brown	----x----

The "x" indicates the over all average of the food group and the dashed line indicates the average range of each food group. Foods in italics contain a large amount of acid and are acid forming for some people and alkaline forming for others, see pages 37 and 41.

	Alkaline ← + neutral – → Acid
	k9 k8 k7 k6 k5 k4 k3 k2 k1 kc0 c1 c2 c3 c4 c5 c6 c7 c8 c9
Rice dream	----x---- (c2)
Rice flour, brown	----x------- (c1)
Rice flour, white	----x---- (c4)
Rice, Japonica	-x------- (k3)
Rice milk	-------x---- (c2)
Rice miso	--------------x------- (k7)
Rice, sweet brown	----x---- (c2)
Rice, sweet brown, pounded (mochi)	----x---- (c1)
Rice syrup, brown	----x------------- (k1)
Rice vinegar, brown (traditional brewed)	----x---- (c1)
Rice, white	-------x-------- (c3)
Rice, wild	----x---- (k1)
Rocambole	----x---- (k4)
Root beer	-----x--- (c6)
Rose hips tea	----x---- (c1)
Rosemary	----x---- (k4)
Rosemary tea	----x---- (k4)
Rutabagas	-----------x----------- (k4)
Rye bread (100%)	----x---- (c2)
Rye bread, organic, sprouted	----x---- (kc0)
Rye bread, refined	----x---- (c3)
Rye crackers, unrefined	-x------- (kc0)
Rye crackers, unrefined, unsalted	-------x-------- (c3)
Rye flakes	-------x-------- (c3)
Rye flour	----x---- (c2)
Rye, whole grain	-------x-------- (c3)
Saccharin	-------x---- (c8)
Safflower oil, cold pressed	--------x----------- (kc0)
Saffron, whole	----x---- (k4)
Sage	----x---- (k4)
Sage tea	----x---- (k4)

The "x" indicates the over all average of the food group and the dashed line indicates the average range of each food group. Foods in italics contain a large amount of acid and are acid forming for some people and alkaline forming for others, see pages 37 and 41.

	Alkaline ← + neutral – → Acid
	k9 k8 k7 k6 k5 k4 k3 k2 k1 kc0 c1 c2 c3 c4 c5 c6 c7 c8 c9
Sake	---------------------------------X----
Sake pickles	-X-------
Salad greens, mixed	----X----
Salami, pork or beef	----X----
Salmon	----X-------
Salsify	----X-------
Salt pickles, using sea salt	----X----
Salt, sea	----X------------------
Salt, table, iodized	-----X----
Salt, table, refined	-----------------------------------X--------
Saltine crackers, with refined salt	----X----
Sapodilla	-X------------------------------
Sapote, white	----X------------------------
Sardines	----X----
Sassafras	----X----
Sassafras bark tea	----X----
Sauerkraut, natural (homemade with sea salt)	---------------X---------
Sausage	-----X----
Sausage, kielbasa	----X----
Sausage, knockwurst, link	----X----
Sausage, pork	----X----
Savory	----X----
Scallions (green onions)	----X-------
Scallops	----X----
Scotch	-----X----
Scrod	----X----
Sea bass	----X----
Sea buckthorn berries	-X-----------------------
Sea palm	----X----
Sea salt	----X------------------

The "x" indicates the over all average of the food group and the dashed line indicates the average range of each food group. Foods in italics contain a large amount of acid and are acid forming for some people and alkaline forming for others, see pages 37 and 41.

	Alkaline ← + neutral – → Acid
	k9 k8 k7 k6 k5 k4 k3 k2 k1 kc0 c1 c2 c3 c4 c5 c6 c7 c8 c9
Sea vegetable powder	----x----
Sea vegetables, most	----x--------
Seeds, canola	----x----
Seeds, chia	----x----
Seeds, flax	-x-----------
Seeds, lotus	----x----
Seeds, most	--------------x-------------
Seeds, pumpkin	----------------------x-----------------------
Seeds, sesame	--------------x----------
Seeds, sesame, black	-----------x------------
Seeds, squash	-----------x-----------------------
Seeds, sunflower	-x------------------------
Seeds, wheat germ	----x----
Seitan (wheat gluten)	----x----
Semolina, sweetened	----x----
Semolina, unsweetened	-------x----
Sesame butter	----------------x-
Sesame oil, unrefined	-----------x-
Sesame salt (gomashio)	----x----
Sesame seeds, black	-----------x------------
Sesame seeds, hulled chemically	----x----
Sesame seeds, hulled mechanically	----x----
Sesame seeds, whole	--------------x----------
Sesame tahini	---------------------x-
Shallots	----x----
Sheep's cheese	---------------x-
Shellfish	----x-----------
Shiitake mushrooms	--------x----
Shiso leaves, fresh or powdered (from making umeboshi)	----x----

The "x" indicates the over all average of the food group and the dashed line indicates the average range of each food group. Foods in italics contain a large amount of acid and are acid forming for some people and alkaline forming for others, see pages 37 and 41.

	Alkaline ← + neutral – → Acid																		
	k9	k8	k7	k6	k5	k4	k3	k2	k1	kc0	c1	c2	c3	c4	c5	c6	c7	c8	c9
Shrimp																X			
Skim milk (non-fat)													X						
Small dried fish															X				
Smelt															X				
Smoothie, banana, unsweetened (fresh fruit only)							X												
Smoothie, fruit, sweetened													X						
Snap beans								X											
Snapper, red																X			
Snow peas						X													
Snow peas, dried						X													
Soba noodles, 100% buckwheat															X				
Soba noodles, 60 to 80% buckwheat																X			
Soft drinks, carbonated																			X
Soldier beans													X						
Sole													X						
Somen noodles, whole wheat														X					
Sorbitol																		X	
Sorghum													X						
Sorghum molasses																X			
Sorrel					X														
Sour cherries									X										
Sour cream													X						
Soy cheese													X						
Soy flour																		X	
Soy grits																X			
Soy hot dogs																X			
Soy ice cream																		X	
Soy margarine															X				
Soy milk, natural and fresh									X										
Soy milk, packaged																		X	

The "x" indicates the over all average of the food group and the dashed line indicates the average range of each food group. Foods in italics contain a large amount of acid and are acid forming for some people and alkaline forming for others, see pages 37 and 41.

	Alkaline ← + neutral – → Acid
	k9 k8 k7 k6 k5 k4 k3 k2 k1 kc0 c1 c2 c3 c4 c5 c6 c7 c8 c9
Soy nuts	`-----x----`
Soy oil	`------------------x----`
Soy protein	`-----x----`
Soy sauce	`----x--------------`
Soy sauce pickles	`----x----`
Soy sauce, processed with sugar and additives	`----x--------------`
Soybean miso	`--------------x-------`
Soybean products, refined (trypsin inhibitor not removed)	`-----x----`
Soybean sprouts	`----x--------`
Soybeans, black	`--------------------x------------------`
Soybeans, dried	`------------------------------x-----------`
Soybeans, green (edamame)	`----x----`
Spaghetti, rye or whole wheat	`----x----`
Spaghetti squash	`----x----`
Spaghetti, white flour	`----x----`
Spearmint tea	`----x----`
Spelt	`-------------x-----------`
Spices, in general	`------------------x-------`
Spinach, cooked	`-------------------------------x-`
Spinach, raw	`----------x-------------------------`
Spiralina	`----x----`
Split peas, green or yellow	`---x--------`
Sprouts, alfalfa	`-------x----`
Sprouts, broccoli	`----x----`
Sprouts, Brussels	`--------------x----`
Sprouts, chia	`----x----`
Sprouts, from amaranth, millet, or quinoa	`--------x----`
Sprouts, from dried soybeans	`----x--------`
Sprouts, from most seeds	`-------x----`

The "x" indicates the over all average of the food group and the dashed line indicates the average range of each food group. Foods in italics contain a large amount of acid and are acid forming for some people and alkaline forming for others, see pages 37 and 41.

	Alkaline ← + neutral – → Acid
	k9 k8 k7 k6 k5 k4 k3 k2 k1 kc0 c1 c2 c3 c4 c5 c6 c7 c8 c9
Sprouts, from other dried beans	-------x-----
Sprouts, from other grains	----x----
Sprouts, radish seed	-------x-------
Squash seeds	--------------x------------
Squash, summer	-----------x----
Squash, winter	-----------x----
Squid	-------x----
Star Anise	----x----
Star fruit	-x-------------------------
Steak	-----x----
Stevia	------------------------------x-----------
Strawberries, sweet	--------------x----------------------
Strawberries, tart	-x------------------
Strawberry tea	-x---------------------
String, green, snap, and wax beans, with formed beans	----x----
String, green, snap, and wax beans, without formed beans	-x-------
Sucanat, dried sugar cane juice (organic), unrefined	----x----
Sucanat, dried sugar cane juice, refined	-------x----
Sucrose	-----x----
Sugar, brown, commercial	-------x----
Sugar cane	-----x----
Sugar cane juice, dried (Sucanat), refined	-------x----
Sugar cane juice, dried (Sucanat), unrefined	----x----
Sugar cane juice, unrefined, evaporated (rapadura)	----x----
Sugar, date	-x-------------------------------
Sugar, maple	----x----

The "x" indicates the over all average of the food group and the dashed line indicates the average range of each food group. Foods in italics contain a large amount of acid and are acid forming for some people and alkaline forming for others, see pages 37 and 41.

Food	Alkaline ← + neutral – → Acid k9 k8 k7 k6 k5 k4 k3 k2 k1 kc0 c1 c2 c3 c4 c5 c6 c7 c8 c9
Sugar, white	-------x---- (c7)
Sulfite (preservative)	----x---- (k4)
Summer squash, crookneck, patty pan, zucchini	----x---- (k5)
Sunflower oil, cold pressed	--------x-------- (kc0)
Sunflower seeds	-x---------------------- (c1)
Sweet brown rice	----x---- (c2)
Sweet brown rice, pounded (mochi)	----x---- (c1)
Sweet brown rice vinegar	----x---- (k3)
Sweet corn (corn on the cob)	----x------- (k4)
Sweet potatoes	-------x---- (k6)
Sweet vegetable drink, mostly root vegetables	----x---- (k5)
Sweet'N Low	-----x--- (c8)
Swiss chard	-----------x----------- (k3)
Swiss cheese	-----------x----------- (c5)
Swordfish	-------x---- (c7)
Tahini	--------------------x- (c4)
Takuwan pickles (daikon)	----x---- (k9)
Tamari, wheat-free	----x-------- (k4)
Tamarillo	----x----------- (k2)
Tamarind	-x------------------------- (k3)
Tangelos	-x------------------------- (k3)
Tangerines	-----------x------------------------- (k3)
Tap water	---x-------- (c1)
Tapioca	----x---- (c2)
Taro potatoes	-----------x----------- (k4)
Tarragon	-------x---- (k4)
Tatsoi	----x---- (k5)
Tea, bancha	----x---- (k4)
Tea, black	--------------x---- (c5)

The "x" indicates the over all average of the food group and the dashed line indicates the average range of each food group. Foods in italics contain a large amount of acid and are acid forming for some people and alkaline forming for others, see pages 37 and 41.

	Alkaline ← + neutral – → Acid k9 k8 k7 k6 k5 k4 k3 k2 k1 kc0 c1 c2 c3 c4 c5 c6 c7 c8 c9
Tea, ginger	-------x-----------
Tea, green	-----------x---------------
Tea, herbal	------------------x----
Tea, mu	--------x----
Tea, red	---x--------
Tea, twig	----x----
Tef	-x-----------
Tekka	----x----
Tempeh	----x-------------------
Thyme	--------x----
Tofu, commercial	-----------x-----------
Tofu, natural nigari	--------x--------
Tomatillo	----x----
Tomato juice	-------x-----------
Tomatoes	----------x------------------
Tortillas, corn	----x----
Triticale	----x-------
Triticale flour	----x-------
Trout	-------x----
Truffles (mushrooms)	----x----
Tuna	----x----
Turban squash	----x----
Turbinado	-------------------x----
Turbot	----x----
Turkey	-----------x-----------
Turkey bologna	----x----
Turkey frankfurters (hot dogs)	----x-------
Turmeric	----x----
Turnip greens	--------x-------
Turnips	--------x-------
Twig tea	----x----

The "x" indicates the over all average of the food group and the dashed line indicates the average range of each food group. Foods in italics contain a large amount of acid and are acid forming for some people and alkaline forming for others, see pages 37 and 41.

Food	Alkaline ← + neutral – → Acid k9 k8 k7 k6 k5 k4 k3 k2 k1 kc0 c1 c2 c3 c4 c5 c6 c7 c8 c9
Udon noodles	(acid side) ----X----
Umeboshi paste	----X----
Umeboshi pickles	----X----
Umeboshi plums	----X--------
Umeboshi vinegar	----X-----------
Urad (like dal)	(acid side) ----X----
Vanilla extract	--------X--------
Veal	(acid side) ------------------X----
Vegetable juice, homemade (no tomato)	-----------X-----------
Vegetable juice, lactofermented	(acid side) ----X----
Vegetable salt	----X----
Veggie burger, mostly bean (other than soy beans)	(acid side) ----X----
Veggie burger, mostly grain	(acid side) ----X-------
Veggie burger, mostly soy	(acid side) -----X---
Venison	(acid side) --------------X--------
Verbena	----X----
Vinegar, acetic	(acid side) -----X---
Vinegar, apple cider, raw, unpasteurized	-------X------------------------
Vinegar, balsamic	(acid side) -------X-----------
Vinegar, brown rice	(acid side) ----X----
Vinegar, red wine	(acid side) -------X----
Vinegar, sweet brown rice	----X----
Vinegar, umeboshi	----X-----------
Vinegar, white, processed	(acid side) --------X---
Vodka	(acid side) -----X---
Wakame	----X----
Walnut oil	(acid side) ----X----
Walnuts, black	-----------X------------------------
Walnuts, English	----------------X--------------------
Wasabi, imitation	----X----

The "x" indicates the over all average of the food group and the dashed line indicates the average range of each food group. Foods in italics contain a large amount of acid and are acid forming for some people and alkaline forming for others, see pages 37 and 41.

	Alkaline ← + neutral – → Acid k9 k8 k7 k6 k5 k4 k3 k2 k1 kc0 c1 c2 c3 c4 c5 c6 c7 c8 c9
Wasabi, true	----X----
Water chestnuts	----X----
Water, filtered	----X----
Water, heavily carbonated	-------X----
Water, in plastic bottle	-------X----
Water, lemon	-X-------------------------------
Water, mineral, heavily carbonated	-------X----
Water, mineral, non-carbonated	----------------------------X-
Water, mineral, slightly carbonated	----X--------
Water, tap (depends on source and how treated)	------------------X--------------------
Water, well	----X----
Watercress	-------X---------------------------
Watermelons	----X--------------------------
Wax beans	----X----
Wheat bran	----X----
Wheat bran cereal	----X----
Wheat, cracked (bulgur)	-------X----
Wheat cream, unrefined	----X----
Wheat flour, white	-----X---
Wheat flour, whole wheat	----X----
Wheat germ seeds	----X----
Wheat gluten (seitan or fu)	----X----
Wheat grass juice	----X----
Wheat, whole	----X----
Wheat, whole, crackers	-------X----
Whey, from cow's milk, fresh	----X--------
Whey, from cow's milk, fully aged	----X----
Whey, from cow's milk, slightly aged	------X--------
Whey, from goat's milk	-------X----
Whey juice, fresh	----X--------

The "x" indicates the over all average of the food group and the dashed line indicates the average range of each food group. Foods in italics contain a large amount of acid and are acid forming for some people and alkaline forming for others, see pages 37 and 41.

	Alkaline ← + neutral – → Acid
	k9 k8 k7 k6 k5 k4 k3 k2 k1 kc0 c1 c2 c3 c4 c5 c6 c7 c8 c9
Whey juice, fully aged	-------x----
Whey juice, slightly aged	------x--------
Whey, protein powder	----x----
Whiskey	-----x---
White beans	---x--------
White bread, yeasted	-----x---
White meat	-----------x-------
White rice	-------x--------
White rice flour	----x----
White sugar	-------x----
White vinegar	-------x----
White wine	----x-------
Whitefish	----x----
Whiting	-------x----
Whole wheat	----x----
Whole wheat bread	----x----
Whole wheat bread, sprouted, organic	----x----
Whole wheat crackers	-------x----
Whole wheat noodles (udon or somen)	----x----
Wild rice	----x----
Wine, red or white	----x-------
Winged beans	----x--------------
Winter squash, most	-----------x----
Wrapped heart mustard cabbage	----x----
Xylitol	-----x---
Yams	----x----
Yannoh	----x------------
Yeast, brewer's or bakers'	----x----
Yeast, commercial	-----x---
Yeast, nutritional	----x----
Yellow beans, with formed beans	----x----

The "x" indicates the over all average of the food group and the dashed line indicates the average range of each food group. Foods in italics contain a large amount of acid and are acid forming for some people and alkaline forming for others, see pages 37 and 41.

	Alkaline ← + neutral – → Acid
	k9 k8 k7 k6 k5 k4 k3 k2 k1 kc0 c1 c2 c3 c4 c5 c6 c7 c8 c9
Yellow beans, without formed beans	----------x----
Yellow bell peppers	-------x-------
Yellow-eyed beans	----x----
Yellowtail	----x----
Yogurt, aged	----x----
Yogurt, dextrogyre	----x----
Yogurt, frozen	-----x---
Yogurt, live culture (levrogyres)	---x--------
Yogurt, plain, fresh	-------x-----------
Yogurt, soy	----------------------x--------------
Yogurt, sweetened	-------x----
Zucchini	----x----

The "x" indicates the over all average of the food group and the dashed line indicates the average range of each food group. Foods in italics contain a large amount of acid and are acid forming for some people and alkaline forming for others, see pages 37 and 41.

References

Acid and alkaline is an evolving field. The first layperson's book on the subject was Herman Aihara's *Acid and Alkaline* (actual title was *Is Acid Yin? Is Alkaline Yang?*) in 1971. Today there are many books on the subject. While there are also a great many websites, be wary of those more interested in selling products than providing information. Here is a brief description of several books for further study.

Acid and Alkaline, 5th Edition – Herman Aihara; George Ohsawa Macrobiotic Foundation; Chico, California; 1986.

While some of the chemical formulas are in an antiquated form and explanations of how to determine acid-forming and alkaline-forming foods can be confusing, the conclusions are as relevant today as when they were written. A large section of the book deals with acid and alkaline compared to yin and yang; this is useful for people who want to study yin and yang or macrobiotics. The book is also useful for people who are interested in only acid and alkaline.

The pH Miracle – Robert O Young, PhD and Selley Redford Young; Warner Books; New York; 2002.

Changes in diet can have a profound effect on one's health and outlook. Dr. Robert O. Young has created an entire dietary program based on his research of acid and alkaline theory. The book contains a full explanation of the theory and the dietary program and it includes many recipes as well. Updates on Dr. Young's work can be found at *www.phmiracleliving.com*.

The Acid-Alkaline Diet for Optimum Health – Christopher Vasey, ND; Healing Arts Press; Rochester, Vermont; 1999.

The explanations of acidity and how to diminish it are clear and the methods of determining excess acidification among the best found anywhere. Another strength of this book is in the chapters of alkaline supplements and methods for draining excess acidity. See Mr. Vasey's website *www.christophervasey.ch* for further information on his activities.

Alkalize or Die – Dr. Theodore A Baroody; Holographic Health Press; Waynesville, North Carolina; 1991.

Theatrics aside, this book is useful for the acid-forming and alkaline-forming values of various foods and for the chapters on lifestyle effects on acid and alkaline. Dr. Baroody is another advocate of the "rule of 80/20"—which means to eat 80% of your foods from the alkaline-forming list and 20% from the acid-forming list. He has developed many products for people needing to alkalize quickly. His website is *www.holisticliving.com.*

The Acid Alkaline Balance Diet – Felicia Drury Kliment; Contemporary Books; New York; 2002.

Professor Kliment clearly explains that acidic wastes are the real culprit behind degenerative disease. After presenting methods for ridding the body of acidic wastes, she gives advice for treating specific ailments. The numerous success stories are particularly engaging. See her website: *www.klimentbooks.com.*

The Acid Alkaline Food Guide – Dr. Susan E. Brown and Larry Trivieri, Jr.; Square One Publishers; Garden City Park, New York; 2006.

Dr. Brown's specialty is bone health, and this book describes the relationship between acid and alkaline and maintaining healthy bones. This book includes chapters on understanding acid-alkaline balance as well as food tables for many foods, including many highly processed foods. Her website is *www.betterbones.com.*

Body Balance – Karta Purkh S. Khalsa, CD-N, RH; Kensington Publishing Corporation; New York; 2004.

Mr. Khalsa is an herbalist who uses pH levels as a way to maintain optimum health. The book includes a useful summary of many natural healing approaches; the bulk of the book is on using various herbs to remedy specific diseases. His website is *www.kpkhalsa.com*.

The New Whole Foods Encyclopedia – Rebecca Wood; Penguin Compass; New York; 1999.

This excellent book provides useful information in "...an alphabetical listing of available grains, vegetables, fruits, nuts, seeds, seaweed, fungi, sweeteners, fats, oils, and culinary herbs and spices." It is highly recommended for anyone interested in whole foods or in using food to improve health. Many articles can be found at Rebecca's website *www.rwood.com*.

Food and Healing, Tenth Anniversary Edition – Annemarie Colbin, PhD; Ballantine Books; New York; 1996.

This book covers all aspects of using food for a healthy life. The part of the book on the dynamics of living systems includes a section on acid and alkaline—highly recommended. Many articles, including one on acid and alkaline, may be found at her website: *www.foodandhealing.com*.

Nature's Cancer-Fighting Foods – Verne Varona; Reward Books; New York; 2001.

This book includes a chapter on acid and alkaline in conjunction with preventing and reversing the most common forms of cancer by choosing the proper foods. Many recipes are included.

A list of books on macrobiotics can be obtained from the George Ohsawa Macrobiotic Foundation, PO Box 3998, Chico, CA 95927-3998; 530-566-9765; 530-566-9768; *gomf@earthlink.net*; or visit *www.gomf.macrobiotic.net*.

Index

Printed in Great Britain
by Amazon